POISONING AND LABORATORY MEDICINE

D1326839

Ian D Watson PhD, FRCPath

Consultant Biochemist, Clinical Laboratories, Aintree Hospitals NHS Trust, Liverpool

Alex T Proudfoot BSc, FRCPE, FRCP

Former Consultant Physician, Royal Infirmary of Edinburgh NHS Trust and Director, Scottish Poisons Information Bureau

Editor:
Roy A Sherwood, M.Sc, D.Phil

Consultant Biochemist, Clinical Biochemistry Department, King's College Hospital, London

ACB VENTURE PUBLICATIONS

with generous support from Dade Behring

ACB VENTURE PUBLICATIONS
Chairman - Roy Sherwood

British Library Cataloguing in Publication Data

A catalogue record for the book is available from the British Library

ISBN 0 902429 30 2 ACB Venture Publications

Printed by KSC Printers Ltd, Tunbridge Wells, Kent

Preface

It is a particularly appropriate time for a book on Clinical Toxicology. Over the past decade or less, major changes in treatment, often evidence based, have occurred. There has been a discernable shift in the poisons encountered in Accident and Emergency Departments. The consequences of these shifts are reflected in the type, frequency and amount of clinical toxicology work demanded of the laboratory. Yet within these changes there are certain basic investigations that need to be performed and a core of poisons, sometimes infrequent, for which detection and/or quantitation can change management. That this is true is attested by the launch of joint guidelines on 'Laboratory Analysis for Poisoned Patients' from the National Poisons Information Service and the Association of Clinical Biochemists. These and the information then current on TOXBASE are reflected in our 'approach', even at the expense of our own opinion! Our aim is for consistency of advice for users of United Kingdom poisons information service.

A distilled UK perspective on poisoning seemed appropriate. It is now nine years since one of us (AP) last published Diagnosis and Management of Acute Poisoning. Many of the texts now available are large or American or both. While estimable the epidemiology, clinical and laboratory approaches are different.

Clinical Toxicology has been taken by us to mean presentation to hospital of a patient, usually with an acute episode. While we recognise the relevance of substance abuse in this context and a short chapter is included, we did not wish undue emphasis on this problem. Similarly forensic, environmental and occupational toxicology are specialist areas in their own right and while briefly mentioned are catered for by specialist texts.

Every endeavour has been made to reflect current thinking on investigation, treatment and even substance names; errors which we hope are few, are however our responsibility.

We are grateful to Michelle Robinson for her energy in ensuring communication between us and efficient document handling, to our editor Roy Sherwood for his efforts and to Richard Hancock and his staff in Medical Photography, University Hospital Aintree for the presentation of the figures.

Ian Watson
Alex Proudfoot
April 2002

ACKNOWLEDGEMENTS

The authors are grateful to the following for permission to reproduce or adapt material for this publication:

The Fine Arts Museums of San Francisco, Achenbach Foundation for Graphic Arts. 1663.30.35055 The Death of Socrates by Daniel Nicholas Chodowiecki (18-19th century) 8.6x11.2cm (image). Cover plate.

ACB Venture Publications. McFarlane I, Bomford A, Sherwood R. *Liver Disease and Laboratory Medicine.* Figure 4.1 p109.

Contents

Chapter 1

Introduction

Only a small proportion of the workload of a hospital laboratory is related to poisoning; of that the vast majority is for a few common requests. A poison may be considered a chemical capable of causing impairment of a living organism; clearly this would be applicable to a wide range of compounds. The circumstances in which a poison is encountered are also significant as they may determine the degree and mode of presentation.

Poisoning is probably as old as mankind; the use of poisonous plants for hunting and assassination is recorded in antiquity. Socrates was forced to commit suicide by ingestion of hemlock (*Conium maculatum*), Romans and their Renaissance successors, the Medici, used poisons for political assassination. The decline of the Roman Empire has been attributed to lead poisoning from their water supply systems. The historical evidence for self-harm by poisoning is less clear, although it undoubtedly occurred.

In the last century or so there have been significant shifts in the causes of mortality (and morbidity) from self-poisoning reflecting the availability of readily utilisable agents. At the beginning of the 20th century phenol (*Lysol*), arsenic and copper sulphate were common poisons, but as legislation was introduced to make them more difficult to obtain and safer replacements became available, their role declined. They were replaced by more readily available chemicals, particularly drugs such as salicylates and barbiturates and also 'town gas' i.e. coal gas containing carbon monoxide. From the early 1970s even these sources declined due to changes in prescribing occasioned by the arrival of new drugs and the replacement of domestic coal gas by natural gas. The commonest poisons now involved in hospital admissions are given in Figure 1.1.

It is perhaps surprising to note the continuing high incidence of carbon monoxide poisoning. This statistic includes not only the victims from fires where carbon monoxide is released but also takes account of suicides, attempted suicides and accidents involving vehicle exhaust emissions and inadequately vented gas appliances in homes. Patients presenting to hospital Accident & Emergency Departments in the UK reflect the relative frequency of different poisonings. However, toxicological analysis does not always confirm the original history and frequently additional drugs are found that may exacerbate symptoms. The commonest additional exogenous compound is ethanol, but benzodiazepines are also common reflecting their ready availability. Figure 1.2 lists the commonest causes of death in descending rank order.

Commonest poisons on admission to hospital*	
Paracetamol	60%
Salicylate	30%
Tricyclic antidepressants and phenothiazines	12%
Ethanol	35%
Carbon monoxide	25%
Others	30%
*Figures are approximate. The total does not add up to 100% as more than one substance may be taken. Ethanol is often consumed in conjunction with drugs.	

Figure 1.1. Commonest poisons on admission to hospital

Commonest poisons implicated in death
Carbon monoxide
Paracetamol
Tricyclic antidepressants
Benzodiazepines
Ethanol
Salicylate

Figure 1.2. Commonest poisons implicated in death (England and Wales)

TYPES OF POISONING

The classification of poisoning is unsatisfactory. It is not based on a single parameter; instead, both the intention behind the incident and its outcome are commonly used. Poisoning can be considered under two main categories, intentional and unintentional and classified as in Figure 1.3. It may also be acute or chronic and the intention may be either acute or chronic.

INTENTIONAL POISONING

SUICIDE
Some individuals deliberately ingest substances with the intention of killing them-

selves. If they succeed they are classified as suicides, but if they fail, they are attempted suicides, parasuicides or self-poisonings, regardless of their expectations. There may be a number of motives for true attempts at suicide including psychiatric illness, e.g. severe depression, and reaction to life circumstances such as loss of family or awareness of illness. Those who truly intend suicide often take measures to ensure that they will not be disturbed; approximately 80% of those who die do not reach medical care. The overall hospital mortality from self-poisoning is less than 1%.

Classification of poisoning	
Intentional	Suicide
	Parasuicide or deliberate self-poisoning
	Substance abuse
	Munchausen's syndrome
	Munchausen's syndrome by proxy
	Homicidal
	Judicial
	Euthanasia
Unintentional	Occupational and environmental
	Iatrogenic
	Accidental

Figure 1.3. Classification of poisoning

PARASUICIDE OR DELIBERATE SELF-POISONING

Parasuicide and deliberate self-poisoning have replaced the term attempted suicide. This is the commonest type of poisoning encountered in adults in developed societies, the peak incidence being in the late teens to about the age of 35 years. The older term was unsatisfactory because it inferred that death was the objective of individuals who deliberately poisoned or injured themselves. Clinical experience indicates that this is not usually the case. Commonly, deliberate ingestion of a poison is an impulsive response at a time of emotional crisis resulting from an accumulation of upsetting and unsettling events. The thought that they might die as a result probably does not cross their minds and, to outsiders, the last straw may seem trivial when considered in isolation. Others indulge in parasuicide to teach someone a lesson or manipulate someone close to them. However, it is usually impossible to know with any certainty the thoughts in the minds of individuals at the moment of action. The depression and psychological hurt at that time may be profound but may pass within hours or even minutes. If they survive, parasuicide is the appropriate classification but if they die, whether or not they intended to do so, they are classified as suicides. The incidence of death and hospitalisation is greater in intentional poisoning even when the subjects expect to survive: their knowledge of the dangers can often be remarkably poor. Ten per cent or more of acute adult medical admissions to hospital in the UK are due to self-poisoning.

SUBSTANCE ABUSE

Some forms of substance use for pleasurable purposes, usually endorsed to varying degrees by the majority, are socially acceptable parts of the cultural milieu e.g. alcohol and tobacco in most countries and the use of cannabis in Rastafarian society. It is then pertinent to consider whether or not consumption that leads to overt toxicity constitutes poisoning or abuse. Substance abuse or misuse is, by definition, unacceptable in law and to the majority of the population, particularly when it is associated with a life style that is dominated by the funding, acquisition and consequences of the use of illegal substances. A small proportion of the population, typically under 30 years of age, misuse substances, including opiates and opioids, amfetamines, cocaine, a variety of 'designer drugs' (e.g. ecstasy) and volatile compounds and sub-populations can often be identified who prefer one class to others. While substance abuse is a deliberate act intended to induce pharmacological effects without risk to life, overdose is an inescapable hazard.

Intravenous injection carries the greatest risk, particularly with drugs such as heroin and morphine (opiates) and their synthetic derivatives (opioids), especially when the purity of the drug supplied increases unexpectedly. In contrast, ingesting and smoking illicit drugs carries a lesser risk of overdose and death. Additional risks run by substance abusers include poor quality products containing toxic by-products, adulterants deliberately added to dilute the drug before sale on the street, and infections if needles are shared.

HOMICIDAL POISONING

Murder by poisoning is rare. Well known instances include the use of ricin (derived from the seed of the castor oil plant) to assassinate a Bulgarian broadcaster, thallium was used by Graham Young to poison his workmates and insulin administration to cause fatal hypoglycaemia in children by Beverley Allitt.

MUNCHAUSEN'S SYNDROME

Adults may consume toxins or injure themselves in other ways to feign medical illnesses that attract attention and sympathy (Munchausen's syndrome). For example, insulin may be used to induce hypoglycaemia and warfarin or anticoagulant rodenticides to induce haematuria.

MUNCHAUSEN'S SYNDROME BY PROXY OR NON-ACCIDENTAL POISONING
Munchausen's syndrome by proxy and non-accidental poisoning are the terms used to categorise cases where for example a child is deliberately poisoned by one of its carers, most commonly its mother. Death is an unusual outcome of this type of poisoning and is not its prime aim. Rather, the perpetrator hopes to attract attention and sympathy through the child's 'illness'.

JUDICIAL
In countries that use the death penalty, lethal injection may be the method used.

EUTHANASIA
In a few countries under tightly defined circumstances death may be assisted by the administration of drugs. This is an area of continuing controversy.

UNINTENTIONAL POISONING
Although unintentional exposure to poisons of any type carries fewer risks than intentional poisoning, significant morbidity and, much less commonly, death may result.

OCCUPATIONAL AND ENVIRONMENTAL POISONING
Poisoning may result from unwitting exposure to chemicals used in manufacturing processes (or the waste products thereof) and may occur either in the workplace or in the wider environment. Occupational and environmental exposure to chemicals is usually chronic and insidious; it is therefore more difficult to diagnose because the exposure/illness relationship may be far from clear or may not be considered by the health professionals involved. In developed countries, industries with known risks e.g. mercury in gauge manufacture, are governed by regulations (in the UK these are set by the Health and Safety Executive on behalf of government ministers). The work place and the workers are monitored regularly to avoid health impairment.

However, acute massive chemical releases are not uncommon. Engineering controls and regular safety checks ensure that they are rare in industry but structural failures occur (e.g. methyl isocyanate in Bhopal), fires in chemical stores lead to explosions and dissemination of complex mixtures of agents and nothing can prevent releases by terrorists (e.g. sarin in Tokyo and Matsumoto). Human error may also result in toxicity (e.g. the accidental addition of a large amount of aluminium salts to the drinking water of the population in the Camelford area of England). The consequences test emergency services to the limit.

IATROGENIC POISONING
Therapeutic errors may result in toxicity and may be considered one end of the spec-

trum of hazards associated with prescribed medicines. Prescription errors can, and do, affect adults, but particular risk is associated with neonates requiring intravenous medication. In these cases the need to calculate doses per kilogram of body weight introduces the potential for miscalculation of both the total amount and the volume of medicine to be administered. Such errors are fortunately rare, but can have devastating physical effects in the recipient and cause emotional turmoil and stress in parents and the staff caring for the child. Pharmacists have a crucial role to play in detecting prescription errors.

Occasionally, inadvertent iatrogenic poisoning may result from failure to recognise impaired function of the principal organ responsible for the elimination of a drug. For example, unrecognised deterioration in renal function may lead to digoxin toxicity in the elderly.

ACCIDENTAL POISONING

CHILDREN

Young children (under the age of three years) are particularly prone to putting objects into their mouths, part of the curiosity of growing up. Indeed, this is the age at which accidental poisoning is most common. Toddlers may be attracted to coloured pills, but also to domestic cleaning agents and other household products of the type commonly kept in cupboards under kitchen sinks. The advent of child-resistant containers has reduced, but not eliminated, the incidence of accidental paediatric poisoning.

ADULTS

At the other extreme of the age spectrum, elderly people may become so confused about the doses of their drugs that they take too much. Confusion and dementia may also cause them to consume other agents such as denture cleaning tablets. However, accidental poisoning is not confined to those in less than full possession of their mental faculties. Mature adults too may inadvertently drink toxic fluids stored in soft-drink bottles e.g. weed killers.

BODY-PACKERS AND STUFFERS

A special type of accidental poisoning in adults is peculiar to those involved in international drug smuggling. They may conceal packets of drugs (commonly heroin or cocaine) amounting to a weight of several kilograms by swallowing them or inserting them into the rectum or vagina to avoid detection by customs officers ('body packing'). Inevitably, rupture of packets and potentially fatal poisoning is a hazard. Others, 'stuffers', consume drugs to avoid being found in possession of illegal substances by the police.

DIRECT (LOCAL) AND SYSTEMIC TOXICITY

While detailed consideration of systemic and local toxicity mechanism is beyond the scope of this text, it is worth remembering that there may be local and systemic effects of a poison.

Toxicity may vary depending on the route of administration. Thus an effective i.v. dose may be an order of magnitude less than a comparable oral dose reflecting poor absorption and hepatic first-pass effects.

DIRECT (LOCAL) TOXICITY

Some toxins directly damage the body membranes with which they come in contact. This is referred to as direct or local toxicity and is independent of any consequences of absorption of the agent into the circulation. Clearly, the temperature of some toxins, e.g. gases inhaled in fires, causes thermal damage to tissues with which they come in contact. Likewise particles in the airways, on the cornea or in the conjunctival recesses of the eye may cause serious irritation, particularly if exposure is lengthy. Similarly, the reaction of strong acids and alkalis with body fluids can produce significant exothermic reactions that add thermal to chemical morbidity.

Direct toxicity of strong acids and alkalis on the mouth, upper gastrointestinal tract, larynx, skin and eye are perhaps the most obvious examples but the inhalation of irritant gases such as ammonia and chlorine, may also damage the respiratory passages and even the alveoli. To some extent, direct damage is a function of the degree of ionisation of the toxin and partly related to its concentration.

SYSTEMIC TOXICITY

Toxicity that is the result of absorption of poisons into the circulation and distribution to tissues is called systemic. Though systemic toxicity may occur without local toxicity and both frequently occur together.

METABOLIC ACTIVATION

Metabolic activation, formerly known as lethal synthesis, is the term used to describe the process by which compounds that are relatively non-toxic in their native state become toxic when they are metabolised. A good example is paracetamol. Less common substances for whose toxicity metabolic activation is a requirement include ethylene glycol, methanol, sodium fluoroacetate and the phosphorothioate group of organophosphate insecticides.

The metabolites of therapeutic doses of paracetamol cause no harm but, when taken in massive overdose, significantly increased amounts of N-acetyl-parabenzo-quinoneimine (NAPQI), a free radical product, are formed. This is normally neutralised by hepatic intracellular glutathione, but after overdose the stores of glutathione are rapidly exhausted allowing NAPQI to cause hepatocellular destruction by reacting with structural thiol groups.

Another example of metabolic activation involving paracetamol has recently been elucidated. Some patients with paracetamol overdoses develop acute renal failure sometimes before significant hepatic damage has occurred. [H]NMR studies have shown that paracetamol is metabolised to p-aminophenol which is nephrotoxic and subsequently conjugated; the p-aminophenol is therefore not identified but is causing toxicity.

Methanol undergoes metabolism to formic acid, ethylene glycol to glycolic, glyoxylic and oxalic acids, fluoroacetate to fluorocitrate and with the phosphorothioates the P=S moiety is converted to P=O, the oxon.

ROUTES OF EXPOSURE TO POISONS

Absorption of poisons may occur by various routes.

INGESTION
In everyday clinical practice ingestion is, by far, the most common route by which poisons are absorbed. Clearly, the proportion of the dose that is absorbed depends on a number of factors. Vomiting induced by the substance may be an important limiting factor if it occurs sufficiently soon after ingestion. Other toxins induce florid diarrhoea and reduce absorption by shortening the gut transit time and some e.g. iron salts and paraquat are inherently very poorly absorbed by the gastrointestinal mucosa. Even so, sufficient may reach the circulation to cause serious toxicity and death.

INJECTION
With two notable exceptions, injection of poisons is uncommon. Intravenous administration ('mainlining') remains the route of choice for some individuals who abuse drugs such as heroin and cocaine, though in recent years a trend involving smoking the drugs has also emerged. The medical literature also contains rare cases where such diverse substances as metallic mercury, organophosphate insecticides, paraquat, insulin and CNS depressant drugs have been injected intravenously. Subcutaneous injection (known as 'skin popping' when involving drugs of abuse) is uncommon but is the usual route for insulin overdoses. Alternatively, intramuscular injection may be used with insulin.

INHALATION

Gases may be innately poisonous or act by diminishing the amount of oxygen available in the air. Inhalation is the commonplace route by which individuals are exposed to the effects of the socially acceptable drug, tobacco and the illegal substances: cannabis, heroin, 'crack' cocaine, volatile substances (solvents/aerosols) and some other substances that are abused. Metals, particularly lead and mercury, can produce acute or chronic systemic toxicity after absorption via this route, most frequently in industrial settings. Health and safety regulations require that concentrations in air are monitored to minimise exposure. Accidental and intentional exposure by inhalation most frequently involves carbon monoxide either in smoke from fires, heating appliances or from vehicle exhaust emissions and is an important cause of deaths from poisoning worldwide.

PERCUTANEOUS

Percutaneous (skin or dermal) exposure to potential toxins is most likely to occur in occupational settings but non-occupational exposures are also possible e.g. when using pesticides in gardens or other chemicals in leisure activities. Absorption is limited by the ability of the substance to penetrate the dermal layer and is increased through damaged skin. In general, lipophilic compounds are more readily absorbed by this route than polar ones and the greater the lipophilicity, the greater the proportion of the dose absorbed. Occasionally, sufficient may reach the circulation to cause systemic toxicity e.g. organophosphates and paraquat. Removal of contaminated clothing and washing the soiled skin with a soap solution are key aspects of management.

OCULAR

Ocular exposure to poisons most commonly results in direct, local injury of the conjunctiva and cornea and usually involves corrosives. However, strong alkalis such as sodium hydroxide may, within only a few minutes, penetrate the deeper structures of the eye causing extensive damage. In such cases it is essential to immediately and continually irrigate the eyes with water for around 30 minutes, having first removed contact lenses if worn and particulate material from the surface of the eye and the conjunctival recesses. Systemic toxicity through ocular exposure is improbable but is recorded, particularly with eye drops containing mydriatics or β-adrenoceptor blocking drugs. Some of the drug passes down the naso-lacrimal duct to the nose where it is absorbed through the epithelium and/or swallowed.

TOXICOKINETICS

The application of pharmacokinetic principles to the poisoned patient is termed toxicokinetics. However, the concept is not always as straightforward as it might seem. The major difficulty with applying standard pharmacokinetic equations to the kinetics of toxic amounts of substances is the lack of reliable data on the dose and time since exposure. Changes in clearance can be easily demonstrated by determining changes in half-life, though zero-order kinetics exhibited by a drug usually exhibiting first-order kinetics is not necessarily predictable between individuals. However, the half-life of some substances is considerably longer after overdose than with therapeutic doses.

Systematic study in man, for example to assess the changes in rate and amount of drug absorbed with and without instillation of activated charcoal, to assess whether there are significant changes in volume of distribution, is nearly impossible. This knowledge, if available, might help in determining the time required for recovery or could be incorporated with toxicodynamic data to produce a predictive model.

The excess of drug taken in overdose may overwhelm clearance mechanisms that cope very well with therapeutic doses; in some cases zero-order kinetics then replace the usual first-order kinetics (e.g. as with theophylline) and there is prolonged exposure to toxic concentrations.

One area that receives some attention, though more is needed, is that of toxin removal by haemoperfusion, haemodialysis and multiple-dose oral activated charcoal. Clearance can be determined for these different treatment modalities and though impressive values may be attained, one of the most notable findings is often how little of the total dose taken has actually been recovered.

CLINICAL PRESENTATION OF THE POISONED PATIENT

DIAGNOSIS
It is always important to establish the history given by the patient, if able, or otherwise by a friend or relative. While unconscious poisoned patients are the exception (no more than 5% of hospital admissions for self-poisoning), many are intoxicated, confused or unresponsive and unsure or unaware of the nature of the drug or poison they have taken. Suicide notes, empty containers or tablets scattered nearby are not uncommon and are particularly helpful. Sometimes drug overdose is only part of a differential diagnosis; it is then important to ensure that early samples are taken for possible subsequent toxicological analysis (see below). The circumstances under which unconscious patients are found: home, workplace, place of entertainment etc., may point to a diagnosis of poisoning. The setting in which the poisoning occurs gives an idea of whether poisoning is intentional, accidental or occupational. Context is a useful contribution to the history. While there may be suspicion of the original cause of any poisoning this does not rule out contribution from other substances, commonly ethanol.

NATURE OF THE POISON: TYPE AND AMOUNT

Tablets and capsules brought with the patient should be examined for size, shape, colour and markings and a Poisons Information Centre or drug information pharmacist contacted to undertake identification. In the UK this is usually done by reference to Tic-Tac, a CD-ROM identification system that also extends to preparations of illegal substances. However, one must always bear in mind that *"the drugs in the hand may not necessarily be the same as those in the patient"*. There is no reliable way of estimating the amount taken; patients' statements about the amounts ingested are generally unreliable since most do not count the number of pills and/or are too far under the influence of alcohol to remember. Occasionally, the amount involved can be estimated from a consideration of the number of unit doses remaining, the date of dispensing (on the container label), the instructions for use (also on the container label) and the number dispensed, the latter being obtained from the pharmacy concerned (also on the container label).

CLINICAL FEATURES

A full clinical assessment of the poisoned patient may reveal combinations of symptoms and signs that may provide clues to the identity of the substance or, at least, lend support to the involvement of specific substances.

NEUROLOGICAL FEATURES

There is commonly evidence of either CNS depression or stimulation which, as with other signs, may provide an indication of the type of poison involved. Scoring systems have been developed to objectively grade the severity of changes in the level of arousal of the brain and to provide baselines from which progress can be assessed. Today, depression of the CNS is usually measured using the Glasgow Coma Score (Figure 1.4) although it was not devised specifically for use in acute poisoning. Systems such as that in Figure 1.5 have also been devised for assessing increased arousal but they are not in general clinical use and have not been validated.

Minor CNS depression may impair muscle co-ordination as manifested by ataxia when walking or nystagmus on movement of the eyes. More severe CNS depression leads to reduced muscle tone and reflexes, reduced respiratory drive, hypotension and impaired body temperature control leading to hypothermia, the degree and rapidity of onset of which is dependent on ambient temperature. In contrast, muscle tone and reflexes are increased by CNS stimulants and intense stimulation may result in severe agitation, motor overactivity, convulsions and hyperpyrexia before coma supervenes.

The Glasgow Coma Score		
Response		**Score**
Eye opening	- None	1
	- To pain only	2
	- To speech	3
	- Spontaneous	4
Verbal response	- None	1
	- Incomprehensible	2
	- Inappropriate words	3
	- Confused conversation	4
	- Normally orientated	5
Motor response	- None	1
	- Abnormal extension (decerebrate rigidity)	2
	- Abnormal flexion	3
	- Withdrawal	4
	- Localised in relation to pain	5
	- Obeys commands	6

The total score ranges from 3-15. A score of 8 or less indicates coma; the lower the score the deeper the coma.

Figure 1.4. Assessment of consciousness – the Glasgow Coma Score (GCS)

Staging increased arousal of the central nervous system
0   Normal
1   Restlessness, insomnia, tachycardia, facial flush, mydriasis
2   As for 1 plus convulsions and mild pyrexia
3   As for 2 plus arrhythmia, delirium, mania, hypertension, hyperpyrexia
4   As for 3 plus convulsions and/or coma

Figure 1.5. Staging increased arousal of the central nervous system

SKIN AND MUSCLE FEATURES
Since unconscious patients lie unmoving, skin blisters can sometimes be seen on the

areas of maximum pressure (note: this is *not* a specific feature of barbiturate poisoning) they should alert the clinician to the possibility of concomitant rhabdomyolysis. Rhabdomyolysis is also a well-documented complication of serious overdosage of CNS stimulants. The presence of needle marks may supply a clue to poisoning by an abused substance.

FEATURES IN OTHER ORGAN SYSTEMS
Figures 1.6 - 1.9 indicate some of the possible explanations for symptoms and signs in the gastrointestinal, respiratory and cardiovascular systems and eyes respectively.

Gastrointestinal features of poisoning	
Feature	**Possible toxin**
Corrosion of lips, mouth and tongue	Strong acids and alkalis Paraquat
Hypersalivation	Organophosphate and carbamate insecticides
Reduced salivation	Anticholinergic agents (e.g. tricyclic antidepressants)
Unusual breath odour	Cyanide (bitter almonds) Chlormethiazole Bleach Phenols and cresols
Dysphagia	Corrosives
Abdominal pain	Corrosives
Diarrhoea	Corrosives and irritants

Figure 1.6. Gastrointestinal features of poisoning

CONFIRMATION OF POISONING AS A CAUSE OF COMA
In the 1960s when barbiturate overdose was a common cause of coma, urgent toxicological analyses were often requested to confirm the diagnosis. However, in developed societies barbiturates are drugs of the past and the common sedatives, tranquillisers and antidepressants involved in poisoning today do not lend themselves so readily to laboratory measurement. Nor would knowledge of their presence or

Respiratory features of poisoning	
Feature	**Possible toxins or mechanisms**
Hypoventilation (reduced depth of respiration)	Depression of the respiratory centre (any agent that impairs consciousness)
Reduction in rate of respiration	Opiate and opioid analgesics
Hyperventilation	Direct effect on the respiratory centre (salicylates, sympathomimetics) Compensation for a metabolic acidosis (salicylate, methanol)
Increased sputum production	Irritants
Cough, breathlessness, wheeze	Irritants (smoke, chlorine)
Aspiration	Petroleum distillates
Pulmonary oedema	Direct lung injury (irritant gases, paraquat, opiate/opioid analgesics)

Figure 1.7. Respiratory features of poisoning

concentrations alter clinical management. Instead, consideration of the symptoms and signs in the context of the circumstantial evidence, available history and knowledge of the patterns of poisoning in the community may provide sufficient information. When poisoning is a high priority in the differential diagnosis of coma, the time to collect samples of blood and urine for confirmation is on presentation and not 24-48 hours later because poisons that are rapidly eliminated may be present only in concentrations that are below the limit of detection of the screening methods commonly used in toxicological analysis by that time.

When considering the differential diagnosis of coma, some information may also arouse suspicion that poisoning is not the cause. Hypoglycaemia can routinely be excluded. Signs of head injury or extensive bruising (not uncommon in overdose patients) may suggest head injury or intracranial bleeding and a CT or MRI brain scan may be indicated. Infectious causes of coma require a similarly high index of suspicion. The progress of an unconscious patient provides an important pointer to the underlying cause. Poisonings usually show significant lightening of coma within 12-24 hours and in cases in which there is no such improvement, another cause is more likely.

Cardiovascular features of poisoning	
Feature	**Possible toxins or mechanisms**
Bradycardia	Cardiac glycosides β-adrenoceptor blocking drugs
Tachycardia	Anticholinergic agents Amfetamines β_2-adrenoceptor stimulants Theophylline
Hypotension	Hypovolaemia (profuse diarrhoea, GI blood loss) Toxin-induced depression of myocardial contractility Acidosis-induced depression of myocardial contractility Tachy- and brady- dysrhythmias
Dysrhythmias	Tricyclic antidepressants β-adrenoceptor blocking drugs β_2-adrenoceptor stimulants Amfetamines Cocaine Theophylline Antiarrhythmic drugs

Figure 1.8. Cardiovascular features of poisoning

BIOCHEMICAL CONSEQUENCES OF POISONING

ACID-BASE DISTURBANCES
Assessment of the arterial oxygen tension, carbon dioxide tension and hydrogen ion concentration is essential for the optimum management of any significantly poisoned patient. If patients have lain undiscovered for sometime they can be hypothermic.

METABOLIC ACIDOSIS
Ingestion of large amounts of an acid or of a compound that is metabolised to an acid will directly result in a metabolic acidosis. Lactic acidosis may be found if anaerobic glycolysis occurs, either as a result of fits, ischaemia or hypovolaemia. Ketoacidosis due to starvation ketosis may be present if the subject has not been found for 24

hours or more; diabetic ketoacidosis may be a possibility in diabetics. A rare syndrome of alcoholic ketoacidosis, usually found in female alcoholics, has significant mortality but is not associated with specific poisoning events.

Ocular features of poisoning	
Feature	**Possible toxins or mechanisms**
Pin-point pupils	Opiate and opioid analgesics Anticholinesterase poisonings (organophosphate and carbamate insecticides)
Dilated pupils	Anticholinergic agents Amfetamines β_2-adrenoceptor stimulants Theophylline Quinine
Nystagmus	CNS depressants Anticonvulsants (particularly phenytoin)
Strabismus	Tricyclic antidepressants and other CNS depressants
Reduced visual acuity	Quinine Methanol

Figure 1.9. Ocular features of poisoning

Ingestion of ethanol results in a mild and usually insignificant metabolic acidosis as a result of metabolism to acidic products. However, metabolism of methanol and ethylene glycol (ethane 1,2 diol) via the same pathways results in strongly acidic metabolites and profound metabolic acidosis. In such poisonings, large amounts of bicarbonate may be required to correct the acidosis. Aspirin (acetylsalicylic acid) as well as being acidic with acidic metabolites, uncouples oxidative phosphorylation contributing a lactic acidosis. Nephrotoxins cause metabolic acidosis due to renal damage.

METABOLIC ALKALOSIS
Uncompensated metabolic alkalosis is a rare event, though it may occur following alkali ingestion. The resultant hypokalaemia may be life threatening. Compensated metabolic alkalosis due to long-term misuse of potassium wasting diuretics or laxatives results in hypokalaemia with consequent metabolic alkalosis.

RESPIRATORY ALKALOSIS

There are two main causes of uncompensated respiratory alkalosis in the poisoned patient, hysteria and direct stimulation of the respiratory centre. Hysteria-induced hyperventilation due to belated concern about drug ingestion can be controlled with re-breathing. Salicylates and CNS stimulants such as theophylline and amfetamines also cause hyperventilation. Direct stimulation of the respiratory centre occurs as salicylate crosses the blood-brain barrier and concentrations increase in the brain; as this passage is enhanced in acidosis this would seem to be at variance with the conventional view that in salicylate poisoning the sequence of acid-base disturbance is respiratory alkalosis followed by metabolic acidosis, however, typically a mixed acid-base picture is seen.

While respiratory compensation to metabolic acidosis will occur, it should be clear from the poison and the biochemistry whether this is compensation or a combined disorder.

RESPIRATORY ACIDOSIS

Reduction in respiratory rate or depth caused by inhibition of the respiratory centre will result in a respiratory acidosis; the cause of which should be clear if a respiratory depressant e.g. opiates have been taken.

ANION GAP

In those clinical biochemistry laboratories in which plasma chloride is offered it is possible to easily calculate the anion gap. In estimation of electrolytes, total CO_2 is not usually measured as part of the profile but bicarbonate is readily derived on a blood gas analyser and will enable the detection of an abnormal anion gap.

The equation:

$$[Na^+] - ([Cl^-] + [HCO_3^-]) = \text{Anion Gap}$$

is recommended; the normal anion gap is 8-18 mmol/L. An alternative form of this equation includes potassium as a cation but as a variation of ± 4 mmol/L for this analyte would be highly clinically significant in itself, it is not relevant to include it in the equation. The change in anion gap caused by the presence of unidentified cations and anions is shown in Figure 1.10.

Presence of an unmeasured cation is a rare situation, but may be seen in lithium poisoning. A far more common situation is one where an increased amount of unmeasured anion is present. If the cause of an increased anion gap is not obvious, measurement of plasma lactate and ketones may help.

Effect of unmeasured cations and anions on the anion gap		
Unmeasured ion present	Anion gap	Explanation
Cation	Low	The sodium contribution to electroneutrality is reduced.
Anion	High	The contribution of measured anions to electroneutrality is reduced.

Figure 1.10. Effect of unmeasured cations and anions on the anion gap

OSMOLAR GAP

The osmolar gap can be used as a very crude screening test to detect whether an osmotically active substance has been taken; the difference between the plasma osmolality measured by freezing point depression is compared with a calculated plasma osmolality. Though a number of different formulae for the calculated osmolality have been proposed, some claiming greater accuracy than others, they are all variations on:

$$2\,[\text{Na}^+]\ +\ [\text{Urea}]\ +\,[\text{Glucose}]\ = \text{Calculated osmolality}$$

where all concentrations are in mmol/L.

A 'normal' osmolar gap is ± 10 mmol/L, therefore this approach is only useful for detecting large changes in osmolality. This calculation is almost exclusively used to obtain a rough approximation of ethanol concentration; it should not be used as a substitute for measurement of ethanol concentrations if action is to be taken on the result and must not be used for other alcohols which are highly toxic at much lower concentrations, though an abnormal osmolar gap would usefully indicate their presence.

PLASMA UREA/CREATININE

As an approximation, pre-renal uraemia, probably due to hypovolaemia, should be suspected if the plasma urea/creatinine ratio (both in mmol/L) is greater than 100. If the substance is a known nephrotoxin then renal function should be checked.

ELECTROLYTES

HYPOCALCAEMIA

Hypocalcaemia following poisoning occurs due to complexation of the circulating calcium. Thus in ethylene glycol poisoning, metabolism leads to large amounts of oxalate being produced which is precipitated as calcium oxalate in tissues and the urine. A similar effect may be seen with phosphates, particularly if they are administered intravenously. Fluoride ions also chelate calcium often causing profound hypocalcaemia and recurrent ventricular fibrillation. Fluoride also chelates magnesium, exacerbating the difficulties in correction of hypocalcaemia.

Drugs such as diuretics and laxatives may cause sufficient magnesium loss to result in inhibition of parathormone release and action and consequent hypocalcaemia.

HYPOKALAEMIA

Hypokalaemia complicating acute poisoning is most commonly the result of redistribution of potassium from the extracellular to the intracellular compartment. It occurs in the presence of an alkalosis or if circulating insulin concentrations are increased, either directly, or indirectly, through catecholamine activity. Hypokalaemia is therefore a common feature in overdoses of insulin, oral hypoglycaemic agents, particularly chlorpropamide (a sulphonylurea with a particularly long half-life) and theophylline (*via* catecholamine release).

HYPERKALAEMIA

Ingestion of potassium salts is rare but can lead to fatal plasma concentrations. While consistent hypokalaemia increases the likelihood of adverse effects of digoxin, particularly at high concentrations of the drug, hyperkalaemia is a sign of significant toxicity in acute digoxin overdose. The rise in plasma potassium is the result of inhibition of membrane Na^+/K^+ ATPase resulting in leakage of potassium from the cells; this has particular relevance as cardiac conduction defects may result in cardiac arrest. Plasma potassium concentrations are also increased when there is release from damaged cells, particularly rhabdomyolysis or haemolysis, and if there is a significant metabolic acidosis.

HYPERNATRAEMIA

Hypernatraemia occurs where there has either been relative water loss or excessive sodium intake, usually as sodium chloride. The outmoded practice of administering salt emetics can cause significant, occasionally fatal, hypernatraemia as can ingestion of bleaches with a high sodium content.

Lithium can induce diabetes insipidus and although this is unusual in acute poisoning, there is a danger of hypernatraemia if saline infusions are given as part of treatment.

Hypernatraemia can occur following infusion of large amounts of sodium bicarbonate to correct profound metabolic acidosis.

HYPONATRAEMIA

Clinically important acute hyponatraemia on presentation is rare in poisoning; when it does occur and is rapid in onset, symptoms of confusion, and coma can result. Hyponatraemia occurs idiosyncratically in some users of 'ecstasy' (3, 4- methylene-dioxy-methamfetamine; MDMA). It can be fatal and is the result of inhibition of vasopressin action exacerbated by drinking water rather than isotonic fluid. More commonly, hyponatraemia is due to compulsive and excessive water drinking, a feature of psychiatric illness.

CHLORIDE

An apparent increase in plasma chloride can be found in bromide poisoning if a ferricyanate method is used.

BLOOD GLUCOSE

HYPERGLYCAEMIA

Patients who have taken substances that stimulate catecholamine release may present with hyperglycaemia due to enhanced glycogenolysis and other anti-insulin actions.

HYPOGLYCAEMIA

Drugs with hypoglycaemic actions, including insulin and sulphonylureas, are obvious causes of overdose-related hypoglycaemia. However, it is also an occasional finding in overdoses of salicylate, ethanol and β-adrenoceptor blocking drugs.

ENZYMES

Changes in plasma enzymes usually reflect the underlying pathological changes as a result of poisoning e.g. raised creatine kinase due to rhabdomyolysis, raised transaminases on late presentation of paracetamol overdose. An exception to this is plasma amylase which may be raised after morphine due to spasm of the sphincter of Oddi. Hyperamylasaemia can occur in paracetamol poisoning raising the possibility that acute pancreatitis is a rare feature of toxicity.

FURTHER READING

GENERAL
Vale JA, Proudfoot AT. Poisoning. Medicine 1999; **27:** 1-58.

Vale JA, Proudfoot AT. Acute poisoning. Concise Oxford Textbook of Medicine. Oxford University Press, 2000.

Gossel TA, Bricker JD. Principles of Clinical Toxicology, 3rd Edition, Raven Press 1994.

Jones AL, Dargan PI. Toxicology. Churchill, Livingstone, London 2001.

EVIDENCE BASED
Buckley NA, Smith AJ. Evidence-based medicine in toxicology: where is the evidence? Lancet. 1996; **347:** 1167-9.

OVERDOSE IN AED
Greaves I, Goodacre S, Grout P. Management of drug overdoses in accident and emergency departments in the United Kingdom. J Accid Emerg Med 1996; **13:** 46-8.

OVERDOSE AND SOCIAL
Smith T. Differences between general practices in hospital admission rates for self-inflicted injury and self-poisoning: influence of socio-economic factors. Br J Gen Pract 1995; **45:** 458-62.

Roberts I, Barker M, Li L. Analysis of trends in deaths from accidental drug poisoning in teenagers, 1985-95, Brit Med J 1997; **315:** 289.

PAEDIATRICS
Bond GR. The Poisoned Child. Evolving concepts in care. Emerg Med Clin North Am 1995; **13:** 343-55.

VOLATILE ABUSE
Flanagan RJ, Ives RJ. Volatile Substance Abuse. Bull Narc 1994; **46:** 49-78.

Sarmiento Martinez J, Guardiola Sala JJ, Martinez Vea A, Campana Casals E. Renal tubular acidosis with an elevated anion in a 'glue sniffer'. Human Toxicol 1989; **8:** 139-40.

CLINICAL TOXICOLOGY
Vale JA. Clinical Toxicology. Postgrad Med J. 1993; **69:** 19-32.

POISONING SEVERITY
Casey PB, Dexter EM, Michell J, Vale JA. The prospective value of the IPCS/EC/EAPCCT poisoning severity scores in cases of poisoning. J Toxicol Clin Toxicol 1998; **36:** 215-7.

SCREENING
Rygnestad T, Berg KJ. Evaulation of benefits of drug analysis in the routine clinical management of acute self -poisoning. J Toxicol Clin Toxicol 1984; **22:** 51-61.

Mahoney, JD, Gross PL, Stern TA, Browne BJ, Pollack MH, Reder V, Mulley AG. Quantitative serum toxic screening in the management of suspected drug overdose. Am J Emerg Med 1990; **8:** 16-22.

Montague RE, Grace RF, Lewis JH, Shenfield GM. Urine drug screens in overdose patients do not contribute to immediate clinical management. Ther Drug Monit 2001 **23:** 47-50.

Carrigan TD, Field H, Illingworth RN, Gaffney P, Hamer DW. Toxicological screening in trauma. J Accid Emerg Med 2000; **17:** 33-7.

Pohjola-Sintonen S, Kivisto KT, Vuori E, Lapatto-Reiniluoto O, Tiula E, Neuvonen PJ. Identification of drugs ingested in acute poisoning: correlation of patient history with drug analysis. Ther Drug Monit 2000; **22:** 749-52.

Steele MT, Westdorp EJ, Garza AG, Ma OJ, Roberts DK, Watson WA. Screening for stimulant use in adult emergency department seizure patients. Clin Toxicol 2000; **38:** 609-13.

Roberts WL, Smith PT, Martin WJ, Rainey PM. Performance characteristics of three serum iron and total iron-binding capacity methods in acute iron overdose. Am J Clin Pathol 1999; **112:** 657-64.

Fitzpatrick R, Hassan T, Ward V, Bodiwala G. Comparison of assays for measuring plasma paracetamol. Training and education in use of assay are important. Brit Med J 1998; **316:** 475-6.

Jones AL, Jarvie DR, Simpson D, Prescott LF. Comparison of assays for measuring plasma paracetamol. Possibility of calibration error needs evaluation. Brit Med J

1998; **316:** 475.

Church AS, Witting WD. Laboratory testing in ethanol, methanol, ethylene glycol, and isopropanol toxicities. J Emerg Med 1997; **15:** 687-92.

Jokanovic M, Maksimovic M. Abnormal cholinesterase activity: understanding and interpretation. Eur J Clin Chem Clin Biochem 1997; **35:** 11-16.

Peredy TR, Powers RD. Bedside diagnostic testing of body fluids. Am J Emerg Med 1997; **15:** 400-7.

Repetto MR, Repetto M. Therapeutic, toxic, and lethal concentrations in human fluids of 90 drugs affecting the cardiovascular and hematopoietic systems. Clin Toxicol 1997; **35:** 345-51.

Repetto MR, Repetto M. Habitual, toxic, and lethal concentrations of 103 drugs of abuse in humans. Clin Toxicol 1997; **35:** 1-9.

Chan TYK, Chan AYW. Use of a plasma salicylate assay service in a medical unit in Hong Kong: a follow-up study. Vet Hum Toxicol 1996; **38:** 278-9.

Glaser DS. Utility of the serum osmol gap in the diagnosis of methanol or ethylene glycol ingestion. Ann Emerg Med 1996; **27:** 343-6.

Liang HK. Clinical evaluation of the poisoned patient and toxic syndromes. Clin Chem 1996; **42:** 1350-5.

Sporer KA, Khayam-Bashi H. Acetaminophen and salicylate serum levels in patients with suicidal ingestion or altered mental status. Am J Emerg Med 1996; **14:** 443-7.

Tomaszewski C, Kirk M, Bingham E, Saltzman B, Cook R, Kulig K. Urine toxicology screens in drivers suspected of driving while impaired from drugs. Clin Toxicol 1996; **34:** 37-44.

Chan TYK, Chan AYW, Ho CS, Critchley JAJH. The clinical value of screening for salicylates in acute poisoning. Vet Hum Toxicol 1995; **37:** 37-8.

CAUSES OF POISONING

McNicholl BP. Toxicity awareness and unintended suicide in drug overdoses. Arch Emerg Med 1992; **9:** 214-9.

Hawton K, Simkin S, Deeks JJ, O'Connor S, Keen A, Altman DG, Philo G, Bulstrade C. Effects of a drug overdose in a television drama on presentations to hospital for self poisoning: time series and questionnaire study. Brit Med J 1999; **318:** 972-7.

TERRORISM

Morita H, Yanagisawa N, Nakajima T, Shimizu M. Sarin poisoning in Matsumoto, Japan. Lancet. 1995; **346:** 290-3.

Chapter 2

Laboratory investigation of poisoning

Routine chemistry parameters such as arterial blood gases, plasma glucose, electrolytes and osmolar gap can help investigation of suspected overdose and may provide a measure of the severity of poisoning (see Biochemical consequences of poisoning p15)

GENERAL CONSIDERATIONS

In a symptomatic patient, knowledge of the presence of a drug may help clarify a differential diagnosis. Intuitively, knowledge of the concentration of a drug may be expected to provide information on the degree of toxicity occurring or to be expected. Indeed, when the establishment of poisons centres was recommended by the Hill Report of 1969 it was anticipated that 'real-time' identification of a drug and knowledge of its concentration would aid patient management. Experience, changing prescribing habits and the introduction of safer drugs have all combined to diminish that expectation. The majority of poisoned patients can be managed supportively and symptomatically without recourse to laboratory toxicology investigations.

Recommendations on 'Laboratory Analyses for Poisoned Patients' were released in 2002 by the National Poisons Information Service and the Association of Clinical Biochemists (NPIS/ACB). These identify those substances for which there should be a 24 hour service and makes recommendations on turnround time for other less common poisons.

TOXIN CONCENTRATIONS

Qualitative analysis enables identification of the poison; this may be time consuming depending on the agent involved. Analysis is commonly performed on urine, though plasma may be used; such analyses are usually retrospective. We use the term plasma but serum may be used as readily. Some estimations require whole blood e.g. for carboxyhaemoglobin, methaemoglobin and metals.

The most frequently requested quantitative toxicological investigations in plasma are salicylate and paracetamol, because these are common, treatable poisonings in which the plasma concentration is related to the severity of toxicity; failure to detect and treat appropriately would be considered to be negligent. There are a very few poisons (around 10 or so) that require quantitation; most of these should be available, at least in a regional laboratory, on a 24 hour a day, 7 days a week basis because effective active intervention is available; they are listed in Figure 2.1. To be relevant other analyses should be available the next day. The NPIS/ACB guidelines give explicit rapid turnround times for some poisons e.g. ethylene glycol and plasma cholinesterase as a marker of organophosphate poisoning which currently most laboratories do not meet.

Poisons for which 24 hour quantitation should be available	
Poison	**Treatment**
Salicylate	Urine alkalinisation Haemodialysis
Paracetamol	N-Acetylcysteine infusion
Lithium	Haemodialysis
Theophylline	Charcoal haemoperfusion
Digoxin	Fab-fragment antibodies
Methanol	Ethanol infusion or fomepizole (4-methylpyrazole)
Ethylene glycol	Ethanol infusion or fomepizole (4-methylpyrazole)
Iron	Desferrioxamine
Phenytoin	Differential diagnosis of convulsions in a known epileptic
Carbon monoxide (as carboxy- haemoglobin; COHb)	Oxygen Hyperbaric oxygen
Ethanol (severe)	Haemodialysis
Methaemoglobin (MetHb)	Methylthioinium chloride (methylene blue)

Figure 2.1. 24 hour availability for quantitative measurement of poisons

Where concentration is a guide to toxicity it may be possible, by making two separate measurements, to determine approximately the poison's half-life thereby obtaining a guide to the probable duration of toxicity. Requests for drug analysis where evidence of a concentration-effect relationship is lacking should be resisted as the additional effort, expense and potential delay are not justified.

TOXICOLOGICAL SCREENING

ACUTE POISONING
In the overwhelming majority of cases toxicological screening adds little to the ability to manage the patient and is only necessary in the circumstances noted below. However when screening has been performed there are often discrepancies between the history given by the patient and the findings of the screen.

A full toxicological screen (usually of urine) may be of value in the differential diagnosis of coma, identifying a cause of unexplained symptoms or in confirming a suspected case of poisoning. Such a screen is a time consuming and expensive process and should not be embarked upon lightly; there has to be a clear clinical benefit from the result.

BRAIN DEATH
A toxicology screen is justified if drugs are thought to be implicated in cases of suspected brain death. If a drug is found, it is necessary to demonstrate its elimination prior to confirming the diagnosis. It is often the case that drugs given therapeutically are detected and have to be proven to be eliminated before brain death can be confirmed.

SITE OF TOXICOLOGY TESTING
Investigation of poisoning is usually performed in the laboratory. However, near patient testing devices may be of help in an Accident and Emergency Department. Breath alcohol meters enable rapid assessment of the contribution of ethanol to symptoms. Reagent sticks for drugs of abuse are particularly useful where symptoms and pharmacological interventions are unclear e.g. for cocaine, amfetamines and methadone poisonings.

METHODS

IMMUNOASSAYS
EMIT and FPIA methods still predominate the available immunoassays and either assay may be used for therapeutic drug monitoring (e.g. theophylline, digoxin) or designed as toxicological screens (e.g. benzodiazepines, tricyclic antidepressants or drugs of abuse).

EMIT (Enzyme Multiplied Immunoassay Technique) is the forerunner of all the readily applicable homogeneous immunoassay methods for drugs. The basic principle is that the antigen/antibody combination inhibits enzyme labelled antibody from catalysing substrate cleavage. The technique is utilisable on common clinical chemistry analysers making it a widely applicable and cost-effective assay for candidate drugs.

FPIA (Fluorescence Polarisation Immunoassay) is a commonly used assay in therapeutic drug monitoring and is also widely used in clinical toxicology. The measurement principle is that bound and free labelled antibody have different rotations in a plane of polarised light, the degree of polarisation being proportional to the amount of drug present.

CEDIA (Cloned Enzyme Donor Immunoassay) is popular for use on general chemistry analysers. An inactive enzyme acceptor associates with a small enzyme donor to form active enzyme. The degree of activity is related to the analyte fraction not bound by the fixed amount of antibody.

A variety of other immunoassays are utilisable, but may not cover the wide range of analytes as the above techniques do as they extend to class screening. There is increasing consolidation of chemistries on clinical chemistry analysers, including therapeutic drug monitoring and clinical toxicology. This is a benefit as 'stat' analyses are more readily performed. Unfortunately, a toxicology panel of barbiturates, benzodiazepines and tricyclics cannot be considered as a definitive screen. Barbiturates are rarely encountered and there may be problems due to differing reactivities of different benzodiazepines or tricyclics. Some potent drugs are therefore missed. Compare this to the drugs identified in Figure 2.1 (p26).

The trend towards common analysers/chemistries can lead to use of expensive immunoassays in place of more specific and cheaper assays e.g. enzymic assay for paracetamol. In 'closed' analyser systems the toxicology/drugs of abuse screening assay is dictated by the instrument manufacturer and the assay performance characteristics may not be adequately documented or available in the literature. Toxicologists must have documented reactivities and interferences for assays used. In certain circumstances detection in an immunoassay system may require chromatographic confirmation e.g. identification of a specific compound where the immunoassay responds to a class of compounds.

CHROMATOGRAPHY

Traditional, classical, toxicological investigation has always had chromatography at its heart. First the drug has to be extracted from the sample matrix, typically urine or serum, and then applied to the chromatography system. Classical methods require investigation of acidic, basic and neutral fractions in a wide-ranging screen for the unknown poison (Figure 2.2).

Extraction of organic drugs from biological fluids	
Liquid/liquid	
Basic compounds	Organic-soluble from basic pH aqueous phase
Acidic compounds	Organic-soluble from acidic pH aqueous phase
Neutral compounds	Organic-soluble
Liquid/solid (reversed-phase)	
Basic compounds	Retain using a basic pH then elute with an acid pH or stronger solvent
Acidic compounds	Retain using an acid pH then elute with an alkaline pH or stronger solvent

Figure 2.2. Extraction of organic drugs from biological fluids

Typically a urine sample is extracted into an organic solvent (e.g. chloroform) from an alkalinised aqueous phase. The organic phase will then contain basic and neutral compounds which may be further 'cleaned up' by back-extraction into an acidic aqueous phase. The aqueous phase after the initial extraction will contain acidic drugs, which can be isolated by making the aqueous phase acidic and extracting into the organic phase.

Liquid-liquid extraction is readily adaptable to a variety of circumstances of polarity, specimen type, volume and concentration of the final extract. This approach is falling into disfavour because of the need to use relatively large volumes of potentially hazardous solvents, the storage and disposal of which is becoming more problematical. Liquid-liquid extraction, while cheap, owes much of its decline to the now widespread use of more expensive, but safer liquid-solid extraction.

Reverse-phase and mixed-bed proprietary phases have extraction schemes that enable reliable isolation of acidic, neutral and basic fractions, although elution may be by aqueous phases necessitating a final concentration step into an organic phase using liquid-liquid extraction. Such schemes are adequate for qualitative analysis, providing there is adequate recovery. If extraction is used to quantify a compound it has been traditional to use an internal standard which is physico-chemically similar to the compound(s) of interest. This serves a dual purpose of providing a reliable retention marker in subsequent chromatography and may also allow correction for extraction losses. Injudicious choice of internal standard can result in increased imprecision due to differences in extraction efficiency between internal standard and the compound of interest.

The three main modes of chromatography are applicable to toxicological investigation.

THIN-LAYER CHROMATOGRAPHY (TLC)

TLC is an ideal method for qualitative investigation for an unknown compound. Compounds may have Rf values (i.e. the distance travelled by the compound of interest relative to the distance travelled by the solvent front) from zero (no elution) to 1.0 (moves with the solvent front).

Silica gel is the commonest adsorbent for 'in-house' systems and the published literature is based on silica gel e.g. methanol/ammonia for basic drug screens. Newer adsorbents are being introduced, but with little impact to date for 'in-house' methods. This probably reflects the large database on the use of silica gels and the absence of data on other systems, particularly for metabolites.

The elution solvents are infinitely variable with minimal methodological restrictions. A frequent strategy is to have an alcohol to ensure solvation and formation of a bilayer on the silica, an anion (or cation as required) for ion suppression and an organic modifier to provide the required polarity e.g. ethyl acetate: ammonia: methanol.

TLC plates are typically glass backed and are run in glass tanks depending on capillary attraction for solvent flow; this can allow solvent de-mixing which can be helpful in achieving certain separations. To increase the resolution of TLC, high performance TLC (HPTLC) is used and, though slightly more expensive, the improvement due to the increased chromatographic efficiency justifies the cost. To achieve discrete application zones calls for a high degree of skill in sample application; satisfactory automated systems are available. Our experience has been that the improved chromatographic efficiency also significantly enhances the lower limit of detection. This may be useful in clinical drug screening where an immunoassay positive result requires confirmation but more sophisticated chromatographic techniques are not available. To achieve this requires attention to technical detail for reliable results. Once a plate has been 'run' and dried the plate must be viewed. Plates containing a fluorescent agent allow the location of compounds when viewed under a UV light as the compounds, as spots, absorb the light.

The plate is then sprayed, or dipped, with location reagent. Some reagents can be applied sequentially causing a series of colour changes. The Rf of the spot and the final colour, or sequence of colour changes, are characteristic of certain drugs or drug classes. This allied to similar information on metabolites helps to characterise the compound. An HPTLC plate of drugs of abuse in urine is shown in Figure 2.3. HPTLC can be analytically sensitive in good hands. TLC is quantitative in conjunction with a good scanning densitometer, the costs of which are comparable to gas chromatography but require the use of specific colour reactions.

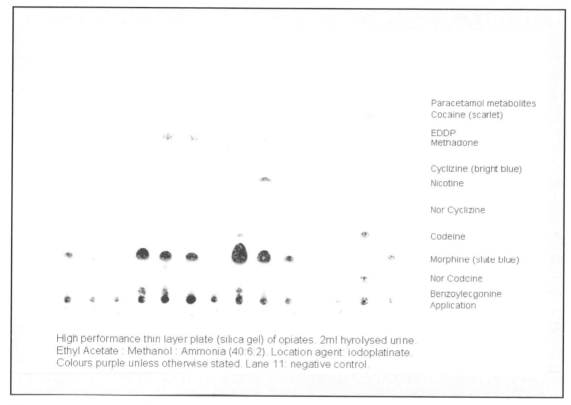

High performance thin layer plate (silica gel) of opiates. 2ml hyrolysed urine. Ethyl Acetate : Methanol : Ammonia (40:6:2). Location agent: iodoplatinate. Colours purple unless otherwise stated. Lane 11: negative control.

Figure 2.3. HPTLC plate of liquid-solid extracted urines for basic drugs of abuse

A commercial TLC system, Toxi-Lab, developed in the USA using a cellulose matrix and the striking colours produced by the Maquis reagent has been very successful in clinical toxicology work. The poor chromatographic efficiency limits sensitivity though this is rarely an issue in overdose. The kit utilises salting-out liquid/liquid extraction for acids or bases with organic solvent evaporation onto a disc of support phase. Following chromatography the Rf and colour changes (± metabolites) are compared to a supplied compendium to enable identification. Although expensive it does allow reliable clinical toxicology screening without the accompanying technical demands. However, its use should not be extended beyond investigation of suspected overdose.

GAS CHROMATOGRAPHY (GC)

Gas chromatography using a capillary column with a flame ionisation detector is an excellent way of detecting and quantifying a wide range of compounds. For improved specificity a nitrogen-phosphorous detector is used. Identification is on the basis of retention time typically based on alkane related retention indices. Such identification is always presumptive and needs corroboration with another non-correlated technique.

Packed column GC is used to identify alcohols, in particular methanol, propanol and ethylene glycol. No other technique is as effective. Figures 2.4 and 2.5 show isothermal chromatograms of methanol, ethanol, acetone, isopropanol, n-propanol (internal standard) and ethylene glycol and propylene glycol (internal standard) respectively. It is of course possible to use a temperature gradient to elute all these alcohols in one run.

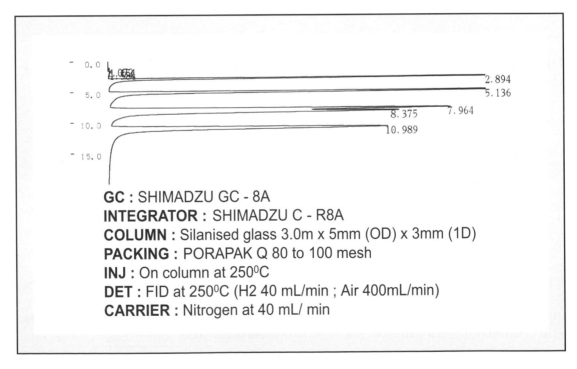

GC : SHIMADZU GC - 8A
INTEGRATOR : SHIMADZU C - R8A
COLUMN : Silanised glass 3.0m x 5mm (OD) x 3mm (1D)
PACKING : PORAPAK Q 80 to 100 mesh
INJ : On column at 250⁰C
DET : FID at 250⁰C (H2 40 mL/min ; Air 400mL/min)
CARRIER : Nitrogen at 40 mL/ min

Figure 2.4. Isothermal GC fid chromatogram of: methanol (2.894), ethanol (5.136), acetone (7.964), isopropanol (8.375) and n-propanol (10.894) [internal standard]

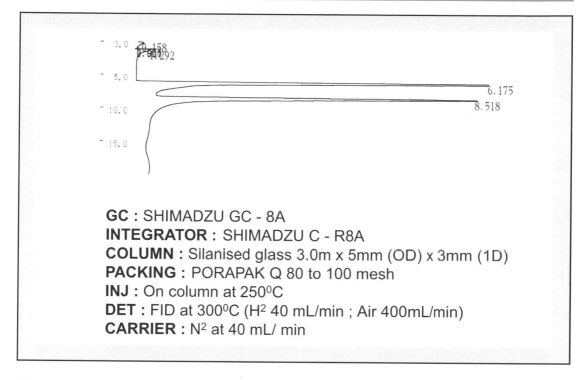

GC : SHIMADZU GC - 8A
INTEGRATOR : SHIMADZU C - R8A
COLUMN : Silanised glass 3.0m x 5mm (OD) x 3mm (1D)
PACKING : PORAPAK Q 80 to 100 mesh
INJ : On column at 250ºC
DET : FID at 300ºC (H² 40 mL/min ; Air 400mL/min)
CARRIER : N² at 40 mL/ min

Figure 2.5. Isothermal GC fid chromatogram of: ethylene glycol (6.175) and propylene glycol (8.518) [internal standard]

Definitive identification by GC can be obtained by using a mass spectrometer (MS) as the detector. Bench-top GC-MS systems are able to provide the retention characteristics, molecular fragmentation (in electron impact mode) and sensitivity (in single ion monitoring mode) that provide definitive proof that a particular compound is present. Best resolution and sensitivity are obtained using sector instruments which are expensive. Adequate performance for clinical toxicology and drug of abuse work is delivered by quadropole or ion-trap MS. Figure 2.6 shows the EI (electron impact) spectrum of 6-monoacetylmorphine.

Figure 2.7 is a total ion current chromatogram of drugs of abuse. There is a requirement for good sample preparation as 'dirty' samples can contaminate the source, internal standards are typically deuterated analogues of the compound(s) of interest. The continual helium purge in some older systems can add significantly to costs.

While most applications use electron impact, some molecules comprehensively fragment making identification of the molecular ion problematic. Alternative methods use chemical ionisation or take a daughter ion from the first MS and pass it through a second electron impact MS (i.e. tandem MS) to obtain characteristic daughter ion fragments. Such sophistication is rarely required in routine clinical toxicology or drugs of abuse work but may be required on occasion.

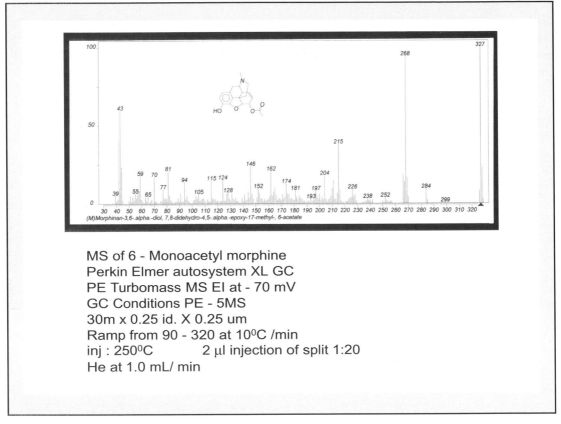

MS of 6 - Monoacetyl morphine
Perkin Elmer autosystem XL GC
PE Turbomass MS EI at - 70 mV
GC Conditions PE - 5MS
30m x 0.25 id. X 0.25 um
Ramp from 90 - 320 at 10°C /min
inj : 250°C   2 µl injection of split 1:20
He at 1.0 mL/ min

Figure 2.6 Electron-impact mass spectrum of 6 mono-acetylmorphine following capillary gas chromatography

National External Quality Assurance returns regularly detect mis-identifications by GC-MS users for drugs of abuse and overdoses. While GC-MS is becoming more common in hospital laboratories it is our belief that where identification is critical samples should be referred to a regional laboratory.

LIQUID CHROMATOGRAPHY (LC)
Typically LC is used to quantify particular analytes rather than for screening. The difficulties in standardising stationary phases for LC has meant that there is variable retention and selectivity for different compounds in such systems. However, linked to a linear diode array detector it has proven possible to obtain a usable screening database. A commercial system with standardised separation conditions and an extensive library of spectra from the linear diode array (LDA) uses comparison of

relative retention and spectra to enable compound identification. This system while popular in the US has not been widely adopted in the UK due to the cost. LC can also be linked to MS but is not routinely used in this way due to expense and technical skill requirements. LC is little used for routine clinical toxicology. Drugs of abuse measurement can be effected by LC but is the exception. LC-MS is being used more frequently for difficult analyses e.g. LSD metabolite detection. This is the preserve of specialist laboratories.

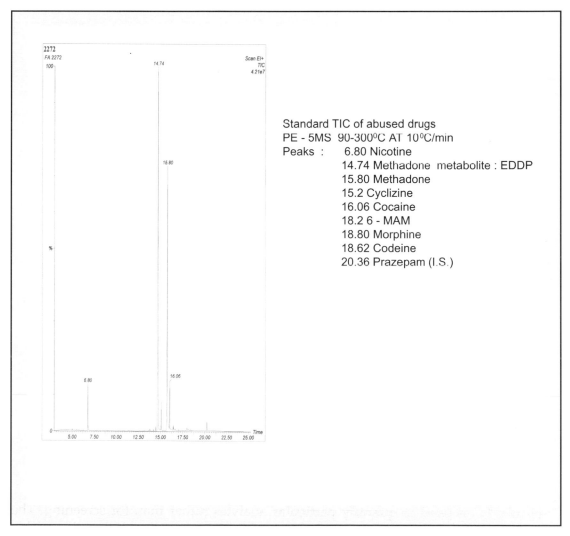

Figure 2.7. GC-MS Total ion-current chromatogram of basic drugs of abuse

The utility of the different modes of chromatography for toxicology are compared in Figure. 2.8

Chromatography for toxicology			
	TLC	**GC**	**LC**
Equipment	Minimal	Expensive	Expensive
Qualitative	Excellent	Good	Moderate
Quantitative	Yes	Yes	Yes
Identification	Good	Poor (excellent with MS)	Very poor (acceptable with LDA) (excellent with MS)

Figure 2.8. Chromatography for toxicology

OTHER TECHNIQUES

Aside from specific analytes (e.g. paracetamol, iron, lithium, salicylate), other screening procedures, now less commonly used but still valuable, are spot urine tests e.g. FPN test for phenothiazines and ultraviolet spectrophotometry, typically of liquid-liquid extracts of urine. Atomic absorption is used to identify particular elements, usually heavy metals.

NEAR-PATIENT TESTING TECHNIQUES

While near patient testing (NPT) is intuitively attractive for clinical toxicology, the wide range of potential drugs and poisons and the lack of difference in clinical intervention that analytical identification makes in the vast majority of cases, has meant NPT has had limited impact. Detection of ethanol, e.g. by breath meters, is frequently used in emergency departments to assess the degree of contribution of ethanol to symptoms. Many stick or cartridge systems are now available for a range of drugs of abuse. While some cartridges cover eight substances, some of the drugs included are so infrequently used in the UK that we prefer discriminatory use of single sticks/cartridges to confirm clinical suspicions. In this scenario identification of the class of compound may be sufficient.

Surprisingly, no acceptable NPT has yet been developed for those compounds requiring quantitation (Figure 2.1, p26), though recently a 'rule-out' device for paracetamol has been reported.

Use of NPT for clinical toxicology has the advantages and problems generally associated with NPT: immediacy versus cost, staff training, result recording etc. Accuracy is a particular problem in toxicology, the NPT devices are usually immunoassay based and therefore prone to non-specificity. Where surveys have been conducted on patients likely to be abusing drugs clinical action has been changed in less than 5% of cases following an NPT analysis. As such tests are available in the laboratory the additional expense associated with NPT does not seem justified.

QUALITY ASSURANCE

Quality assurance in clinical toxicology can be difficult to achieve. For some common drugs there are quantitative schemes, for drugs of abuse qualitative schemes and in some cases schemes offered for therapeutic drug monitoring will suffice. Similarly internal quality control materials will be available. However, clinical toxicology potentially extends over a wide range of exogenous compounds. For many there are no guaranteed pure materials nor metabolites. The UKNEQAS schemes cover therapeutic drug monitoring, drugs of abuse and clinical toxicology. UKNEQAS has recently introduced a toxicology case scheme combining the requirement for analysis and interpretation. Laboratories providing toxicological analyses should be members of the appropriate schemes.

Quality Assurance surveys have demonstrated inappropriate analytical procedures giving qualitatively and/or quantitatively erroneous results. Extension of the schemes into interpretative case scenarios has revealed a wide spectrum of abilities.

For analytes where no scheme exists, there is no quality control nor is there good reference material, probably these analyses would best be referred onward to an expert laboratory.

IDENTIFICATION OF SUBSTANCES

A systematic approach to investigation needs an extraction strategy to extract a wide range of compounds from the sample followed by chromatography, preferably using two modes in which the physio-chemical basis of separation has a low correlation (e.g. GC and TLC with location agents). For a compound to be identified with around 90% certainty it will extract into a particular fraction (e.g. basic), display appropriate chromatographic retention on both chromatography systems and give the appropriate colour reactions with the TLC location reagent. The security of the identification is improved if metabolites with appropriate chromatographic and chemical behaviour are also found. The findings have to be allied to the history and clinical information.

When a screen is conducted it is not uncommon to find that substances other than that first suspected are found. The laboratory has a duty to inform the clinician of all substances found even if these might be drugs, such as lignocaine, which may have been administered by medical staff. The commonest additional substance in a poisoning is ethanol.

Results of toxicological screens should be discussed with the clinician concerned. The laboratory staff should have the required expertise to provide an informed assessment of the findings in relation to the patient's condition and to be aware of any problems with methods used or further analyses that could be helpful.

Clinical toxicology is an opportunistic specialty in the sense that people poison themselves in a variety of novel ways and a single case report that is well documented can help others confronted with a similar problem. Systematic study of types and presentations of poisoning is often difficult because there are too few cases. The National Poisons Information Service are linked to reference centres for such types of study, being able to bring expert knowledge and skills to bear and co-ordinate information on the investigations and treatment of unusual poisonings.

Opportunities for toxicokinetic studies should be sought. Good toxicokinetic studies are difficult to conduct, requiring a balance between effective patient management, ethics and co-ordination between the treating physician and the toxicology laboratory.

SAMPLE TYPES

Concentration-effect relationships, where established, are performed on plasma (or serum). Screening may be performed on plasma/serum but more commonly urine is used because it has a higher concentration of the unknown substance and/or its metabolites, and is available in greater volumes, making detection and identification easier.

Gastric contents may contain undigested or partially digested tablets or capsules which may identify the poison taken. As gastric lavage is now less frequently performed this information may be lost. Analysis of gastric contents is rarely rewarding. Saliva can be tested for ethanol using a strip device.

INTERPRETATION

Advice is readily available from the NPIS. This service has recently been reorganised so that each of its components has regional responsibilities. All Accident and Emergency staff make regular use of the NPIS which holds up to date information on a wide variety of drugs, plants, household and industrial substances. An information scientist usually gives advice initially but access to specialist medical advice is available in some centres. Advice is also accessible by subscription to TOXBASE, an NPIS web-based service. This is available free of charge to health professionals (www.spib.axl.co.uk) or by telephone (0870 600 6266). Enquirers must access TOXBASE before telephoning NPIS. For a few common poisonings there are established treatment guidelines that are readily usable by competent clinical and laboratory staff. As a rule, laboratory staff who are not experienced in toxicology should not give advice on the significance of laboratory toxicology results and treatment of poisoning.

FURTHER READING

LABORATORY SUPPORT
Clarke's Isolation and Identification of Drugs in pharmaceuticals, body fluids and post-mortem material. 2nd Edn. Eds. Moffat AS, Jackson JV, Moss MS, Widdop, B. The Pharmaceutical Press: London 1986 [New Edition in preparation]

LABORATORY SUPPORT FOR THE POISONED PATIENT.
Watson ID. Laboratory support for the poisoned patient. Ther Drug Monit 1998; **20:** 490-7.

Badcock NR. Detection of poisoning by substances other than drugs: a neglected art. Ann Clin Biochem 2000; **37:** 146-57.

National Poisons Information Service and Association of Clinical Biochemists. Joint Position Paper: Laboratory Analyses for Poisoned Patients. Ann Clin Biochem 2002; In Press.

QUALITY ASSURANCE
Wilson JF, Toseland PA, Capp NE, Sandle LN, Smith BL, Sweeney G, Thomson AH, Watson ID, Williams J. External quality assessment of laboratory performance in analysis of toxicological cases. Forensic Sci Int 2001; **121:** 27-32.

Watson ID, Wilson JF, Toseland PA, Smith BL, Williams J, Capp NE, Thomson AH, Sweeney G, Sandle LN. Scoring and performance of analysis and interpretation of toxicologic cases assessed by external quality assurance. Ther Drug Monit 2002; **24:** 156-8.

Chapter 3

Treatment options in poisoning

EMERGENCY MEASURES

While most patients overdosing on drugs show few symptoms or signs, those who are severely poisoned require rapid, effective intervention to maintain life; in these cases treatment centres on the maintenance of vital functions. Application of the ABC of resuscitation:

- Airway
- Breathing
- Circulation

is the initial imperative (Figure 3.1).

The ABC of resuscitation

Airway:
- ensure there is no blockage of the airway
- no obstruction by the tongue
- no loose dental plates (remove if necessary)
- no vomit or saliva in the oropharyngeal area

Breathing:
- assess ventilation adequacy (arterial blood gases)
- spontaneous respiration if appropriate
- appropriate ventilatory support as required

Circulation:
- maintain an adequate circulation
- determine the cause of hypotension
- correct hypoxia and also respiratory and/or metabolic acidosis
- monitor the central venous pressure
- use appropriate inotropic agents if necessary

Figure 3.1. The ABC of resuscitation

GENERAL PRINCIPLES – THE IMPORTANCE OF SUPPORTIVE CARE

It is important to realise that once satisfactory vital functions have been stabilised in acutely poisoned patients, the vast majority are likely to survive provided these functions are adequately maintained until such times as the toxin is eliminated. This process has long been known as supportive care and monitoring of arterial blood gas tensions and renal and liver function with routine clinical biochemistry tests is essential to its success. Supportive care also aims to minimise the impact of secondary contributions made by partially blocked airways and inadequate ventilation and circulation. It is imperative that any treatment additional to supportive care must reasonably be expected to reduce the morbidity from poisoning and/or shorten the time to recovery; ideally, it should not add to either, though use should not be withheld if risk assessment is in favour of benefit. The supplementary measures that are peculiar to acutely poisoned patients include antidotes (if available), and techniques to minimise absorption and distribution of the toxin or maximise its rate of elimination.

OBTAIN INFORMATION ABOUT THE POISON

Knowledge of the toxicity of the substance or how to manage poisoning with it informs carers of the complications that might arise and the rough time course of events. It is, therefore, a highly desirable pre-requisite for optimum clinical management. Some substances are ingested so commonly that their toxicity is well known. However, if there is uncertainty, it is advisable to obtain information at an early stage, initially by accessing TOXBASE, the computerised, primary toxicology database of the UK NPIS. On-line registration is available at the web address of the database:

http://www.spib.axl.co.uk

Alternatively, one of the centres in the NPIS can be contacted directly for this information. Unfortunately, data are not always available for rare poisons, but something of help is usually offered. Complicated poisonings may be best managed in consultation with the NPIS, although there is no legal requirement for this.

ANTIDOTES

A number of antidotes are available for use in clinical toxicology. They are listed in Figure 3.2 together with the toxins against which they are effective and their modes of action. N-acetylcysteine (*Parvolex*) is by far the most commonly used followed by naloxone (*Narcan*). In developed societies the patterns of acute and chronic poisoning are such that the other antidotes find only a sporadic role.

Use of antidotes		
Substances	**Action**	**Agent**
Metals	Chelation	Calcium sodium edetate Desferrioxamine Dimercaprol Succimer (dimercaptosuccinic acid; DMSA) Unithiol (dimercapto-1-propane sulphonate; DMPS)
Methanol and Ethylene glycol	Competitive inhibition of metabolism	Ethanol Fomepizole (4-methylpyrazole)
Paracetamol	Substrate supplementation	N-Acetylcysteine Methionine
Opiates/opioids	Competition for receptors	Naloxone

Figure 3.2. Use of antidotes

MINIMISING ABSORPTION

It would seem sensible to try to minimise absorption of poisons from the gut (gastrointestinal or gut decontamination) and over the years a number of methods have been used. Some of them, such as the use of strong salt or copper sulphate solutions to provoke emesis, are, or should be, of no more than historical interest, but they still may be encountered as 'folk memory' brings them into play. Methods that are, or were, in use until very recently, include ipecacuanha-induced vomiting, gastric lavage, administration of adsorbents, cathartics and whole bowel irrigation. However, the value of gut decontamination procedures has long been controversial and, in an attempt to make the management of acute poisoning more evidence-based, the American Academy of Clinical Toxicology (AACT) and the European Association of Poisons Centres and Clinical Toxicologists (EAPCCT) have critically reviewed the evidence for their use and published the outcome in the form of position statements. If implemented, their recommendations should reduce the workload of carers and protect patients from unnecessary invasive, disagreeable and degrading experiences. Restriction of access to the more toxic substances is an effective option, this covers a spectrum from a ban on production through tight prescription control to restricting pack size and packaging in blister packs.

GASTRIC EMPTYING BY INDUCED EMESIS

Attempting to empty the stomach by inducing emesis is no longer considered useful, regardless of the age of the patient or the method used. In particular, syrup of ipecacuanha is relegated to the past. Its active ingredients, emetine and cephaeline, may have induced vomiting consistently and rapidly (within 20 minutes in 80% of those given it), but there was no evidence that it altered the course of poisoning. Indeed, in many cases features attributed to the poison may well have been due to the treatment.

GASTRIC EMPTYING BY LAVAGE

Gastric lavage, not for the first time, has also been the object of criticism. The theory behind its use may appear rational, but in practice there is very little evidence that it alters the course of poisoning for the better. Its use also carries dangers including aspiration of saliva and gastric contents into the lungs, the induction of hypoxia and tachycardia (which may exacerbate impaired cardiac function when a cardiotoxic poison has been taken) and, rarely, perforation of the oesophagus. Equally important, there is also evidence that the procedure may force gastric contents beyond the pylorus, increasing the absorption of toxin and rapidly increasing the severity of poisoning. It has, therefore, been recommended that the use of gastric lavage should be *considered* only when:

- a significantly toxic amount of a substance has been swallowed and
- the procedure can be performed within one hour of ingestion.

These recommendations beg definition of what constitutes 'a significantly toxic amount of a substance' and that is an issue yet to be addressed. However, if followed, there should be a significant decline in the use of lavage. Clearly, even when performed soon after ingestion, lavage is only warranted if the patient's airway can be protected. It is carried out by instilling around 250 mL (in adults) of tepid tap water (to avoid hypothermia) into the stomach, mixing the stomach contents by massage over the upper abdomen and then draining, repeating this procedure until the fluid returned is clear. Even then there is a possibility that concretions of drugs may not have been dislodged or dissolved. Absolute contraindications to gastric lavage include ingestion of strong acids and alkalis; ingestion of long chain hydrocarbons (petroleum distillates) is a relative contraindication.

SINGLE-DOSE ORAL ACTIVATED CHARCOAL

The greater use of adsorbents is expected to replace gastric emptying techniques, for the immediate future at least. While a number of adsorbents such as kaolin and

Fullers' earth have been tried over the years, activated charcoal is the only practical option. Charcoal has been known from the beginning of the 19th century to be effective in neutralising poisons and it will undoubtedly be used more widely.

The process of activating charcoal involves heating the source material to a high temperature in a stream of gas which oxidises and greatly increases the surface area of the charcoal particles, potentially up to 3,500 m^2/g. Activated charcoal has no direct pharmacological effects, yet it is capable of adsorbing a wide range of poisons. In general, it is most effective in adsorbing organic compounds and as with gastric emptying techniques, is most effective if given early after poisoning. Indeed, it is probably of no value in reducing absorption if it is given later than one hour after ingestion. In the UK there are currently five licensed preparations: *Actidose-Aqua*, *Carbomix*, *Charcodote*, *Liqui-Char* and *Medicoal*. The usual initial dose is 25-100 g for an adult, 25-50 g for children aged 1-12 years and 1g/kg body weight for children under the age of one year. Unfortunately activated charcoal is not a panacea. Evidence of its efficacy in clinical situations is scant and it does not adsorb inorganic ions, alcohols, petroleum distillates, strong acids or alkalis or organic solvents. More importantly, patient acceptability is low and limits its usefulness. Some formulations are black, unappetising in appearance and administered as slurries that leave an unpleasant gritty feel in the mouth. Attempts to disguise these attributes have had very limited success. Nausea is a common adverse effect of oral charcoal administration and the soiling of individuals and surroundings can be considerable when patients vomit. Constipation is another side effect which, in rare, severe cases, can result in intestinal obstruction.

CATHARTICS
No data are available to indicate that the outcome of acute poisoning is improved by giving cathartics. The AACT and EAPCCT have, therefore, concluded that they have no role in management.

WHOLE BOWEL IRRIGATION
A potentially effective approach to minimising absorption of some poisons is the use of whole bowel irrigation (WBI), but evidence of efficacy is very limited. The consensus view is that, if valuable at all, WBI is likely to be of greatest benefit in the management of patients who have ingested potentially toxic amounts of sustained release or enteric coated drug formulations that have already passed into the small bowel and continue to be absorbed. These are most likely to comprise iron salts and theophylline preparations. WBI has also been advocated for decontaminating body-packers. Irrigation is performed using proprietary solutions of polyethylene glycol and electrolytes, such as *GoLytely* and *Klean-Prep,* that claim to effect good recovery with minimal clinical and biochemical problems, even in infants and in pregnancy.

ELIMINATION TECHNIQUES

A variety of techniques have been used to enhance the rate of elimination of toxins from poisoned patients.

FORCED DIURESIS

From the 1950s until comparatively recently, forced diuresis was used widely in the management of a variety of poisonings, particularly salicylate intoxication and commonly in conjunction with measures to alkalinise the urine. However, defining the relative merits of diuresis and alkalinisation of the urine has long been a problem not addressed by early clinical studies. Forced diuresis had the advantage of requiring neither special equipment nor expertise. On the other hand, it was inadequately defined in terms of the rate of urine flow to be attained or the time for which diuresis was to be sustained. Instead, an arbitrary amount of fluid was given intravenously over a relatively short period of time (e.g. 6L over three hours for salicylate intoxication in adults).

Forced diuresis can only enhance the elimination of poisons that are reabsorbed from the renal tubular fluid and acts by speeding urine flow thus reducing the time the toxin spends in the renal tubule and the time available for reabsorption. However, studies in poisoned patients have shown that any reduction in plasma salicylate concentrations induced by forced diuresis was simply the result of haemodilution rather than enhanced urinary excretion. Many patients with salicylate intoxication were slow to increase their rate of urine production in response to forced diuresis with the result that fluid overload and pulmonary oedema developed. The technique was also used in a number of situations where present day knowledge of the kinetic properties of the toxin made it highly improbable that it could have been of benefit. The indications for forced diuresis have therefore been severely restricted by the AACT and EAPCCT. Indeed, its only indication may be for poisoning with chlorophenoxy herbicides and, only then, in conjunction with urine alkalinisation.

MANIPULATION OF URINE pH

Manipulation of urine pH, alkalinisation for weakly acidic (salicylates, phenobarbital) and acidification for basic compounds (amfetamines, phencyclidine), was one of the first elimination techniques to be soundly based on pharmacokinetic principles. The rationale is that the change in urine pH increases ionisation of the drug thus impairing its re-absorption from the renal tubular fluid. In practice today, the use of urinary alkalinisation as an elimination technique is almost entirely confined to the treatment of poisoning with salicylate and the chlorophenoxy herbicides 2,4-D (2,4-dichlorophenoxyacetic acid), mecoprop (MCPP or 2-(4-chloro-2-methylphenoxy)propionic acid) and dichlorprop (DCPP or 2-(2,4-dichlorophenoxy)propanoic acid). The usual approach is to give 1.5 L of 1.26% sodium bicarbonate intravenously over three hours. Urine pH should be tested at intervals; a pH approaching 8.0 is desirable. Hypokalaemia and hypocalcaemia are potential complications if urinary alkalinisation is continued over a protracted period (as formerly occurred in phenobarbital intoxication). The alkalaemia induced does not appear to carry adverse effects.

In contrast, urinary acidification (achieved by infusing a solution of ammonium chloride intravenously) has never found a significant clinical role and that remains the case today; it should not be used. Poisonings in which it might be effective can be managed satisfactorily in other ways.

DIALYSIS
Peritoneal dialysis and haemodialysis can be used to enhance the elimination of toxins that are hydrophilic, have a low molecular weight (<350 Daltons) and, preferably, a small volume of distribution. Although haemodialysis is the method of choice because it is about four times more efficient than peritoneal dialysis, the latter still has a valuable therapeutic role in geographically remote regions lacking facilities for immediate haemodialysis. In reality, in developed societies neither technique is frequently used to increase the rate of elimination of poisons. Dialysis is indicated in severe poisoning with salicylates, lithium, potassium salts, methanol, ethylene glycol and chlorophenoxy herbicides, all of which are rare. When a poison has a large volume of distribution, a rebound increase in its plasma concentration can be expected shortly after discontinuing haemodialysis.

CHARCOAL AND RESIN HAEMOPERFUSION
Charcoal haemoperfusion was introduced into clinical toxicology by a Greek physician in the early 1960s. Resin haemoperfusion arrived later. Both are carried out in a way similar to haemodialysis. Arterial blood is led from the patient to the bottom of a column containing activated charcoal or resin which adsorbs drug present in the blood. Once it has traversed the column the blood is then filtered and returned to the patient. These techniques are particularly apposite for severe poisoning with lipophilic substances that cannot readily be removed by dialysis. Unfortunately for the manufacturers of charcoal and resin cartridges, acute barbiturate poisoning, the situation in which they could have made a major clinical impact, had largely disappeared by the time columns became commercially available; they now have virtually no role. Transient thrombocytopenia is a well-described complication of their use.

MULTIPLE DOSE ORAL ACTIVATED CHARCOAL – 'GUT DIALYSIS'
The concept of gut dialysis was introduced about 15 years ago when it was demonstrated that repeated doses of oral activated charcoal significantly shortened the plasma half-life of phenobarbital given intravenously to volunteers. Multiple-dose

charcoal was later shown to be of considerable benefit in acute poisoning with this drug and has the inestimable advantage of reducing toxicity without resort to sophisticated techniques. The mechanism of action is thought to be as follows. The charcoal in the gut lumen acts as a sump, binding drug and ensuring a near zero concentration of the drug in the luminal fluid. This creates a concentration gradient that promotes the movement of drug from the blood flowing through the microscopic superficial vessels in the microvilli of the gut mucosa to the lumen, thus reducing blood concentrations and body load. The dose of charcoal for an adult is 100g given 4 hourly or smaller doses correspondingly more frequently until charcoal appears in the faeces.

Drug poisonings for which there is evidence for the efficacy of multiple-dose charcoal are listed in Figure 3.3. There are others for which the evidence is controversial e.g. phenytoin, salicylates. The NPIS will advise on the appropriateness of the use of multiple-dose charcoal in individual patients.

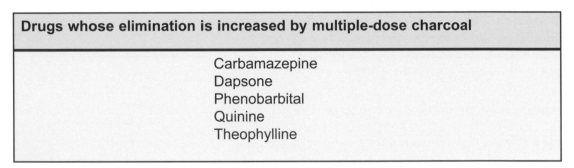

Drugs whose elimination is increased by multiple-dose charcoal

Carbamazepine
Dapsone
Phenobarbital
Quinine
Theophylline

Figure 3.3. Drugs whose elimination is increased by multiple-dose charcoal

CONCLUSION

The management of acute poisoning requires a more thoughtful approach than has been apparent in recent decades. Fortunately, seriously poisoned patients will undoubtedly receive the optimum supportive care they need; it is the prime requirement. It is the use of treatment options specific to acute poisoning – gut decontamination, antidotes and elimination techniques – that will continue to cause controversy and anxiety. Interventions of these types, however well intentioned, are not necessarily of value or safe, and knee-jerk therapeutic responses to clinical problems cannot be condoned in the absence of evidence of efficacy. The vast majority of individuals exposed to potential poisons will not develop features of toxicity and, therefore, do not require treatment. Many patients with symptoms will not warrant active intervention. Gastric lavage and/or a single dose of oral activated charcoal may be useful if performed or administered within one hour of ingestion but it is inevitable that single-dose charcoal will be used to bind poisons for which there is no evidence that it is effective. Urine alkalinisation should be used for toxins whose elimination is amenable to enhancement by it. The indications for the use of multiple-dose oral activated charcoal, dialysis and charcoal haemoperfusion to enhance the elimination of toxins are well defined. Many previously accepted manoeuvres – emesis, cathartics and forced diuresis – are no longer acceptable.

FURTHER READING

AVAILABILITY
Robinson D, Smith AMJ, Johnston GD. Severity of overdose after restriction of paracetamol availability: retrospective study. Brit Med J 2000; **321:** 926-7.

INDUCED EMESIS
American Academy of Clinical Toxicology and European Association of Poisons Centres and Clinical Toxicologists. Position statement: Ipecac syrup. J Toxicol Clin Toxicol 1997; **35:** 699-709.

GASTRIC LAVAGE
American Academy of Clinical Toxicology and European Association of Poisons Centres and Clinical Toxicologists Position statement: Gastric lavage. J Toxicol Clin Toxicol 1997; **35:** 711-9.

ACTIVATED CHARCOAL
American Academy of Clinical Toxicology and European Association of Poisons Centres and Clinical Toxicologists Position statement: Single-dose oral activated charcoal. J Toxicol Clin Toxicol 1997; **35:** 721-41.

American Academy of Clinical Toxicology and European Association of Poisons Centres and Clinical Toxicologists Position statement: Multiple-dose oral activated charcoal. J Toxicol Clin Toxicol 1999; 37: 731-51.

CATHARTICS
American Academy of Clinical Toxicology and European Association of Poisons Centres and Clinical Toxicologists Position statement: Cathartics. J Toxicol Clin Toxicol 1997; **35:** 743-52.

WHOLE BOWEL IRRIGATION
Whole Bowel Irrigation. American Academy of Clinical Toxicology and European Association of Poisons Centres and Clinical Toxicologists Position statement: Whole bowel irrigation. J Toxicol Clin Toxicol 1997; **35:** 753-62.

Chapter 4

Poisoning with specific substances

Advice in this section is as far as possible, consistent with UK practice. Contact the National Poisons Information service for latest advice.

β₂-ADRENOCEPTOR STIMULANTS

IMPORTANT FACTS
- Salbutamol and terbutaline are the members of this group of drugs that have been most commonly encountered in overdose.

- Overdose with fenoterol, pirbuterol, reprobuterol or rimiterol would be expected to cause similar effects.

- Poisoning has followed deliberate and accidental ingestion of these drugs.

- Poisoning may also result from confusion over the difference between oral and parenteral doses.

MECHANISM OF TOXICITY
- Direct stimulation of the central nervous system.

CLINICAL FEATURES

Clinical features of poisoning with β-adrenoceptor stimulants	
Common	**Uncommon**
Excitement	Convulsions
Hallucinations	Ventricular tachycardia
Agitation	Pulmonary oedema
Palpitations	
Tachycardia	
Tremor	

LABORATORY FEATURES
- Hypokalaemia.

- Hyperglycaemia.

- Lactic acidosis.

PLASMA CONCENTRATIONS
- Are of no value in the management of acute overdose.

MANAGEMENT
- Gastric lavage for patients who present within one hour of ingestion of a substantial overdose or a single dose of oral activated charcoal may be given.

- Correct hypokalaemia with intravenous potassium (40 to 60 mmol/h in 5% dextrose).

- If potassium is given, beware rebound hyperkalaemia during recovery.

- Propranolol (1-5 mg by slow intravenous injection) also reverses β_2-stimulant-induced hypokalaemia; care is required since it may exacerbate pre-existing obstructive pulmonary disease.

AMFETAMINES AND ECSTASY

IMPORTANT FACTS
- Amfetamine and 'ecstasy' (3,4-methylenedioxymethamfetamine, MDMA) are the amfetamines most commonly seen in clinical practice.

- Dexamfetamine and methamfetamine are seldom encountered.

- The vast majority of individuals who use these drugs, intermittently or regularly, do not develop significant acute toxicity. There is evidence that sustained use results in long-term diminution of cognitive function.

MECHANISM OF TOXICITY
- Direct stimulation of the central nervous system.

CLINICAL FEATURES

Clinical features of poisoning with amfetamine or ecstasy	
Common	**Uncommon**
Euphoria	Paranoia
Increased alertness	Violent behaviour
Increased self-confidence	Convulsions
Extrovert behaviour	Cardiac arrhythmias
Rapid, increased speech	Hypotension
Loss of appetite	Coma
Loss of need for sleep	Hyperpyrexia
Tremor	Rhabdomyolysis
Dilated pupils	Intracranial haemorrhage
Tachycardia	Cardiomyopathy
Hypertension	Vasculitis
	Acute hepatic necrosis

LABORATORY FEATURES
- Metabolic acidosis.

- Raised creatine kinase activity.

- Increased hepatic transaminase activity.

- Hyponatraemia secondary to inappropriate ADH secretion may complicate ecstasy use.

- Hyperthyroxinaemia may be found in chronic users.

PLASMA CONCENTRATIONS
- Are of no value in the management of acute overdose.

- Urine screens for amfetamines may fail to detect metamfetamines and vice versa.

MANAGEMENT
- Gastric lavage for patients who present within one hour of ingestion of a substantial overdose or a single dose of oral activated charcoal may be given.

- Sedation may be required.

- β-adrenoceptor blocking drugs can be used to antagonise the peripheral sympathomimetic actions of amfetamines.

- Acidification of the urine increases the renal elimination of methamfetamine five-fold but should be seldom, if ever, necessary.

- Other symptomatic measures.

ANTICOAGULANTS

IMPORTANT FACTS

- Warfarin is the most widely used oral anticoagulant and the one most commonly involved in accidental and therapeutic overdoses. Rarely, phenindione may be encountered.

- Accidental poisoning is most common in young children and due to eating mouse and rat baits.

- The newer and widely used anticoagulant rodenticides, brodifacoum, bromodiolone, chlorophacinone, coumatetralyl, difenacoum and flocoumafen are considerably more potent than warfarin.

- Surreptitious ingestion presenting with bleeding has been reported in adults.

- Management is more complex when overdose occurs in patients who are anticoagulated because of prosthetic heart valves.

MECHANISM OF TOXICITY

- Synthesis of vitamin K_1 from its biologically inactive metabolite, vitamin K_1 2,3-epoxide, is inhibited leading to reduced concentrations of factors II, VII, IX and X.

CLINICAL FEATURES

- Bruising, haematuria and gastrointestinal bleeding are the usual presenting features.

- Intracranial haemorrhage is the most common cause of deaths.

LABORATORY FEATURES

- Prolongation of the prothrombin time or International Normalised Ratio (INR).

- A single dose of an anticoagulant rodenticide, other than warfarin, may significantly impair clotting for weeks or months.

- Orange coloured urine (not due to blood) may be seen after phenindione overdose.

PLASMA CONCENTRATIONS

- Are of no relevance to the management of the overdose.

MANAGEMENT
- Gastric lavage is not indicated.

- A single dose of oral activated charcoal or cholestyramine may be given to adsorb anticoagulant remaining in the gastrointestinal tract.

IF CONTINUING ANTICOAGULATION IS NOT REQUIRED, THE INR IS GREATER THAN 6, OR BLEEDING HAS OCCURRED
- Give vitamin K_1 (phytomenadione), 5 mg , slowly, intravenously.

IF CONTINUING ANTICOAGULATION IS REQUIRED AND THE PATIENT IS NOT BLEEDING
- Stop the warfarin if the INR is less than 8.

- If the INR is >8 give Vitamin K_1 (discuss the dose with coagulation experts or haematologists).

- Re-start warfarin when the INR has fallen to an acceptable value (usually <5).

IF CONTINUING ANTICOAGULATION IS REQUIRED AND SERIOUS BLEEDING IS PRESENT
- Prothrombin complex concentrate (50 units/kg body weight) and Vitamin K_1 may be required.

- Fresh frozen plasma (15 mL/kg body weight) may be used if prothrombin complex concentrate is not available.

- Consult with coagulation experts or haematologists.

IF PROLONGED, UNNECESSARY ANTICOAGULATION OCCURS
- Give oral phytomenadione.

BENZODIAZEPINES

IMPORTANT FACTS

- Benzodiazepine overdose is common, though less so than it was some years ago.

- Benzodiazepine overdose alone is rarely fatal.

- Benzodiazepines are toxicologically important because they potentiate the CNS depressant effects of other drugs including tricyclic antidepressants, opiates and opioids and ethanol.

- Their anticonvulsant activity may be an advantage when they are taken in conjunction with overdoses of other drugs that induce convulsions, e.g. tricyclic antidepressants.

- The metabolites of some benzodiazepines are toxicologically active.

MECHANISM OF TOXICITY

- Benzodiazepines depress the central nervous system.

CLINICAL FEATURES

Clinical features of poisoning with benzodiazepines	
Common	**Uncommon**
Drowsiness	Coma
Slurred speech	Respiratory depression
Unsteadiness	Hypothermia
Mild hypotension	Skin blisters
Nystagmus	

LABORATORY FEATURES

- Mild reduction of PaO_2 and increase in $PaCO_2$.

PLASMA CONCENTRATIONS

- Are of no value in the management of acute overdose.

- Quoted concentrations may include active and inactive metabolites in addition to parent drug.

MANAGEMENT
- Gastric lavage is unnecessary unless an adult has ingested more than 30 therapeutic doses within the previous hour.

- Supportive measures as indicated by the patient's clinical state.

- Consider giving the specific benzodiazepine antagonist flumazenil (0.5 mg intravenously over 30 seconds) for severe poisoning. If necessary, the same dose may be repeated. A total dose of 1-3 mg will usually reverse toxicity completely.

CARBAMATE INSECTICIDES

IMPORTANT FACTS
- Carbamate insecticides act in the same way as organophosphate (OP) insecticides (see p103).

- Carbamate insecticides are readily absorbed through the gut, respiratory tract and skin.

- The features of poisoning with carbamates are very similar to those of OP poisoning.

- Carbamate poisoning is generally less severe and of shorter duration than OP poisoning because spontaneous reactivation of carbamate-inhibited cholinesterase is relatively rapid.

MECHANISMS OF TOXICITY
- Carbamate insecticides inhibit acetylcholinesterase in the brain, at peripheral nerve endings and in ganglia in the autonomic nervous system.

- The speed of onset, severity and duration of toxicity caused by individual carbamates vary considerably and depend on a number of factors.

- High tissue concentrations of insecticide and high affinity of the enzyme for it increase toxicity.

- The faster the insecticide-enzyme complex hydrolyses (thus 'reactivating' the enzyme) the less is the intensity and the shorter is the duration of poisoning.

- The carbamate-enzyme complex does not undergo 'ageing' as do OP's (see below).

CLINICAL FEATURES
It is customary to classify the features of poisoning by cholinesterase inhibitors into muscarinic and nicotinic. The latter occur mainly at neuromuscular junctions. Muscarinic features usually occur first and in the alimentary or respiratory tract depending on which is the route of exposure. Respiratory failure is the usual cause of death and results from a combination of depressed respiratory drive, weakness of the respiratory muscles, airways obstruction secondary to bronchospasm and retention of bronchial secretions. Severe poisoning may also be complicated by convulsions, coma and cardiac arrhythmias.

Clinical features of poisoning with carbamate insecticides	
Muscarinic	**Nicotinic**
Anxiety	Fasciculation
Restlessness	Increasing muscle flaccidity and/or muscle
Dizziness	weakness (including the external eye muscle
Salivation	and the muscles of respiration)
Tear production	
Bronchorrhoea	
Bronchospasm	
Abdominal colic	
Urgency of micturition	
Urgent bowel movements	
Sinus bradycardia	

LABORATORY FEATURES
- Red cell cholinesterase (acetylcholinesterase) and plasma cholinesterase (pseudo-cholinesterase or butyryl cholinesterase) activities are both reduced.

CHOLINESTERASE ACTIVITY
The diagnosis can be confirmed by demonstrating reduced plasma or, preferably, erythrocyte cholinesterase activity. Cholinesterase activity is commonly in the range:
- 50-70% of normal in asymptomatic patients
- 10-20% in moderate poisoning
- less than 10% in severe poisoning.

MANAGEMENT
- Further absorption from dermal exposure will be reduced by removing soiled clothing.

- Gastric lavage should be considered for patients who present within one hour of ingestion of a substantial amount.

- Supportive measures should be implemented as necessary and are of paramount importance.

- Atropine can be used but is less commonly required than in organophosphate poisoning since carbamate intoxication is usually short-lived.

- The use of oximes e.g. praladoxime is unnecessary in the vast majority of cases as spontaneous reactivation of inhibited enzyme occurs comparatively rapidly.

CARBAMAZEPINE

IMPORTANT FACTS

- Carbamazepine overdose may be therapeutic or due to intentional self-harm.

- Carbamazepine is most likely to be taken in overdose by epileptics and those taking the drug as part of a pain relief regimen.

- Carbamazepine is chemically and toxicologically similar to the tricyclic antidepressants.

MECHANISM OF TOXICITY

- The mechanism is not understood.

CLINICAL FEATURES

Clinical features of poisoning with carbamazepine	
Common	**Uncommon**
Drowsiness	Respiratory depression
Nystagmus	Paralysis of the external eye muscles
Ataxia	Choreiform movements
Dilated pupils	
Increased muscle tone	
Violent reactions to being roused	
Hallucinations	
Divergent squint	
Convulsions	

LABORATORY FEATURES

- None of note.

PLASMA CONCENTRATIONS

- Therapeutic concentrations are within the range 0-10 mg/L (0-45 μmol/L).

- Measurement of serum carbamazepine concentration is useful for confirming over- and under-dosage.

- The plasma half-life of the drug after overdosage is considerably longer than with therapeutic doses.

- Plasma concentrations are important in deciding when to re-start regular treatment in an epileptic who has been poisoned with carbamazepine.

MANAGEMENT
- Gastric lavage for patients who present within one hour of ingestion of a substantial overdose.

- Supportive measures are usually all that are required.

- Multiple-dose oral activated charcoal shortens the plasma half-life of carbamazepine.

CARBON MONOXIDE

IMPORTANT FACTS

- Carbon monoxide (CO) poisoning may be acute, subacute, chronic or occult.

- CO is one of the most important causes of deaths from poisoning in many developed countries.

- Vehicle exhaust fumes and smoke from fires are the commonest sources of CO.

- Badly installed domestic gas heating appliances and incomplete combustion of butane and propane (e.g. in caravans) may lead to subacute, chronic or occult poisoning.

- Rarely, exposure to methylene chloride (commonly used as a paint stripper) may lead to carbon monoxide poisoning.

MECHANISMS OF TOXICITY

Haemoglobin has an affinity for CO some 200-300 times greater than it has for oxygen. Most of the toxic effects of CO can therefore be explained by reduced oxygen delivery to tissues.

- The combination of CO with haemoglobin to form carboxyhaemoglobin (COHb) reduces the oxygen-carrying capacity of the blood.

- The formation of COHb shifts the oxyhaemoglobin dissociation curve to the left impairing liberation of oxygen to cells.

- Oxygen binding sites are altered in such a way that the affinity of the remaining haem groups for oxygen is increased thus impairing oxygen liberation in the tissues.

- CO binds to myoglobin and cytochrome oxidases (especially cytochrome a and cytochrome a_3) and may impair the ability of tissues to utilise the oxygen they receive.

- Impaired tissue oxygenation may be exacerbated by hypotension, particularly in vulnerable organs such as the brain.

- Developing fetuses are also at increased risk because their normal arterial oxygen tension is low (about 30 mm Hg 4 KPa) and because their oxyhaemoglobin dissociation curve, normally to the left of that of the mother, will be further shifted to the left.

CLINICAL FEATURES - ACUTE POISONING

Immediate features of carbon monoxide poisoning	
Common	**Uncommon**
Headache	Rhabdomyolysis
Dizziness	Myocardial infarction
Nausea	Pulmonary oedema
Drowsiness leading to coma	Retinal haemorrhages
Features of acute gastroenteritis	Cerebral oedema
Hyperventilation	Skin blisters
Hypotension	Parkinsonism
Increased muscle tone	Chorea and choreo-athetosis
Hyper-reflexia	Cortical blindness
Cyanosis (the cherry-pink skin	Mutism
colour that is considered to be	Hemiplegia
classical of this form of	Peripheral neuropathy
poisoning is seldom seen)	

DELAYED NEUROPSYCHIATRIC SEQUELAE
Some patients (usually adults over the age of 40 years) who appear to recover completely from acute poisoning develop symptoms and signs of CNS white matter damage days or weeks later. The clinical consequences include apathy, disorientation, amnesia and hypokinesia. Urinary and/or faecal incontinence, irritability, easy distractibility, apraxia, and behavioural abnormalities also occur but are less common.

ACUTE POISONING IN PREGNANCY
Fetal hypoxia and death is the likely outcome. Animal studies suggest that the COHb concentration in the fetus probably increases slowly to reach a level that is 10-15% higher than that of the mother.

CLINICAL FEATURES – SUBACUTE, CHRONIC AND OCCULT POISONING
These include common and non-specific symptoms such as:
- headache
- dizziness
- fatigue
- general malaise

- a flu-like feeling.

A high index of suspicion is required if the correct cause is to be identified.

LABORATORY FEATURES
- Metabolic acidosis.

- Normal oxygen tension but reduced oxygen saturation.

- Features of organ damage e.g. kidneys, skeletal muscle.

CARBOXYHAEMOGLOBIN CONCENTRATIONS
- Elevated COHb concentrations confirm the diagnosis.

- A COIIb concentration of 20% or more has been proposed as an indication for hyperbaric oxygen therapy, the relevance of COHb concentrations is an area of controversy.

- Smokers may have COHb concentrations up to 8%.

- Non-smoking, city dwellers may have COHb concentrations up to 5%.

- The finding of an increased COHb concentration in alleged subacute or chronic poisoning is important and has legal implications.

- Fetal COHb disappears more slowly than the mother's once exposure has ceased.

- Due to the greater prevalence of cardiovascular disease in the elderly there is increased morbidity and mortality associated with carbon monoxide poisoning.

MANAGEMENT
- The patient will have been removed from the toxic atmosphere by the emergency services.

- Supportive measures to ensure a clear airway and adequate ventilation and blood pressure are vital.

- Initially, the inspired oxygen concentration should be increased as far as possible, using a tight-fitting face mask.

- Assisted ventilation may occasionally be required.

- Correct metabolic acidosis by ensuring optimum oxygenation and, if appropriate, reducing increased muscle activity using dantrolene. Avoid giving alkali – it may further impair oxygen release to tissues through its effect on the oxyhaemoglobin dissociation curve.

- Avoid excess fluid administration.

- Give mannitol and dexamethasone if cerebral oedema is present.

- Consider referral for hyperbaric oxygen (HBO) treatment if poisoning is clinically severe, there has been loss of consciousness at any time after exposure, neurological or psychiatric features are present, the patient is pregnant or COHb concentrations exceed 20%. HBO (a common protocol involves two hours or longer at 2-3 atmospheres) improves oxygen delivery to cells by increasing the amount of oxygen dissolved in plasma and shortening the half-life of COHb from about 250 minutes when breathing air to 25 minutes. However, despite its apparent logic, controlled trials have not shown HBO to be of value. Until the situation is clarified by further studies, the appropriateness of HBO referral should be discussed with the National Poisons Information Service.

CARDIAC GLYCOSIDES

IMPORTANT FACTS

- Digoxin is by far the most commonly used cardiac glycoside in the UK. Digitoxin is rarely encountered.

- Therapeutic overdose of these drugs is much more common than intentional overdose.

- Acute poisoning with digoxin and digitoxin is infrequent but carries a mortality as high as 20%.

- Plants such as the foxglove, some species of oleander and yew contain cardiac glycosides or chemicals with similar actions.

MECHANISM OF TOXICITY

- Cardiac glycosides inhibit the cell membrane Na^+-K^+ pump.

CLINICAL FEATURES

Clinical features of poisoning with cardiac glycosides	
Common	**Uncommon**
Nausea	Ventricular premature beats
Vomiting	Supraventricular arrhythmias
Dizziness	Ventricular tachycardia
Drowsiness	Peripheral circulatory failure
Confusion	
Diarrhoea	
Visual disturbances	
Hallucinations	
Sinus bradycardia (often marked)	
First degree heart block	

LABORATORY FEATURES

- Hyperkalaemia occurs due to inhibition of the Na^+ - K^+ activated ATPase pump.

- A metabolic acidosis may be present.

PLASMA CONCENTRATIONS

- Diagnosis is confirmed by measuring plasma digoxin concentration, but concentrations correlate poorly with toxicity in acute poisoning.

- Concentrations can be used to calculate the total body burden of digoxin or digitoxin and thus the amount of antidote required.

- Treatment with Fab fragments results in interference in digoxin assays.

- Cardiac glycosides other than digoxin react variably in digoxin immunoassays.

MANAGEMENT
- Gastric lavage for patients who present within one hour of ingestion of a substantial overdose.

- A single dose of oral activated charcoal may reduce absorption.

- Potassium supplements should not be given until the serum potassium concentration is known. Hyperkalaemia should be managed conventionally.

- Correct metabolic acidosis.

- Atropine may reduce or abolish sinus bradycardia, ventricular ectopics, atrio-ventricular block and sino-atrial arrest or block.

- Ventricular ectopic beats alone do not require treatment unless cardiac output is impaired.

- Lignocaine, atenolol, phenytoin or amiodarone may be used to treat ventricular tachydysrhythmias.

- In severe poisoning the use of ovine Fab-fragment anti-digoxin antibodies (6-8 mg/kg body weight) should be considered; they should produce improvement in about 30 min.

- Cardiac pacing is indicated if the above measures fail to achieve a satisfactory cardiac output.

- Elimination techniques of any type are of little value; they have been superseded by digoxin-specific antibodies.

- Multiple-dose oral activated charcoal may enhance elimination of cardiac glycosides.

CHLORATES

IMPORTANT FACTS
- Serious chlorate poisoning is very uncommon.

- Chlorates are highly toxic if ingested.

MECHANISM OF TOXICITY
- Sodium and potassium chlorate are powerful oxidising agents.

CLINICAL FEATURES
- Nausea, vomiting, diarrhoea and abdominal pain are the typical initial features.

- Later, cyanosis secondary to methaemoglobinaemia develops.

- Intravascular haemolysis may follow leading to hyperkalaemia, jaundice, and oliguric renal failure.

LABORATORY FEATURES
- The blood may be chocolate-brown in colour if significant methaemoglobinaemia is present.

- The plasma and urine may have a brownish colour caused by the presence of haemoglobin that has been released from damaged erythrocytes.

- Blood films may show red cells containing Heinz bodies (denatured globin adherent to the inner surface of the cell membrane).

- Early hyperkalaemia is likely to be the result of haemolysis.

- Later hyperkalaemia is due to the onset of acute renal failure.

- Hyperbilirubinaemia develops after 12-24 hours and is secondary to increased production from damaged red cells.

PLASMA OR BLOOD CONCENTRATIONS
- There are no data on plasma chlorate concentrations in acute chlorate poisoning.

- Measurement of the blood methaemoglobin concentration may be useful in identifying patients who should be given the antidote.

MANAGEMENT

- Gastric lavage for patients who present within one hour of ingestion of a substantial amount.

- Monitor plasma potassium concentrations and, if indicated, treat hyperkalaemia.

- Correct methaemoglobin concentrations in excess of 20% by slow intravenous injection of methylthioninium chloride (methylene blue; 2 mg/kg body weight as a 1% solution).

- Blood transfusion may be required, but is preferably delayed until the chlorate has been cleared from the body.

- Haemodialysis removes chlorate, but criteria for its use have not been established.

- Renal failure should be managed conventionally.

- Plasmapheresis has also been advocated to remove circulating free haemoglobin and red cell stroma in addition to chlorate. This may help prevent the development of renal failure.

COCAINE

IMPORTANT FACTS
- Cocaine misuse is now common and increasingly affordable.

- Cocaine (cocaine hydrochloride) is typically 'snorted' but is also used intravenously, sometimes in combination with heroin. 'Crack' cocaine (cocaine base, i.e. cocaine without the hydrochloride moiety) is smoked.

- Topical application of cocaine solutions is occasionally employed in surgery, partly because of its local anaesthetic properties, but more often because it results in a blood-free surgical field.

- Cocaine is teratogenic.

- Body packing is a common method of smuggling cocaine.

MECHANISMS OF TOXICITY
- Cocaine blocks the uptake of catecholamines at adrenergic nerve endings, potentiating their actions. It is, therefore, initially a CNS stimulant; high doses cause CNS depression. It causes intense vasoconstriction.

- Neurochemically cocaine affects dopamine and 5-hydroxytryptamine transmission and may also affect corticotrophin releasing hormone release.

Clinical features of cocaine poisoning	
Common	**Uncommon**
Euphoria	Headache
Agitation	Delirium
Sinus tachycardia	Convulsions
Hypertension	Hyperpyrexia
Tachypnoea	Rhabdomyolysis
Sweating	Coma
Ataxia	Ventricular dysrhythmias
Dilated pupils	Myocardial infarction
Hallucinations	Cerebral infarction
	Subarachnoid haemorrhage
	Hypokalaemic paralysis
	Premature labour and fetal death

In addition, cocaine misusers are at risk of complications specific to the route and duration of administration including pneumothorax and pneumomediastinum from smoking, pulmonary oedema from intravenous use, bacterial and viral infections from needle sharing, and nasal septum perforation, cerebrospinal fluid rhinorrhea and lung granulomas from snorting.

LABORATORY FEATURES
- Metabolic acidosis

- Hypokalaemia

- Hyperkalaemia and raised creatine kinase activity when rhabdomyolysis occurs.

PLASMA CONCENTRATIONS
- Are of no value in the management of cocaine poisoning.

MANAGEMENT
- Establish a clear airway and ensure adequate oxygenation.

- Assist ventilation if necessary.

- Monitor the ECG.

- Control convulsions with diazepam; muscle paralysis, endotracheal intubation and mechanical ventilation may be required if status epilepticus persists.

- Treat metabolic acidosis that persists after control of convulsions and correction of hypoxaemia with intravenous sodium bicarbonate.

- Persistent hypertension may require the use of intravenous glyceryl trinitrate or calcium antagonists; avoid using beta-adrenoceptor blockers.

- Implement measures to counteract hyperthermia, including giving dantrolene if body temperature exceeds 39°C.

- Complications such as rhabdomyolysis, ventricular dysrhythmias, myocardial ischaemia and cerebral infarction are managed conventionally.

- Features of cocaine toxicity in any cocaine body packer indicates that some of the packets are leaking; urgent surgery to remove them is indicated.

ETHANOL

IMPORTANT FACTS
- Ethanol intoxication is extremely common in adults and an increasing problem in young teenagers.

- Some 60% of men and 40% of women who deliberately take drug overdoses will have consumed alcohol before or at the same time.

- Ethanol is an important antidote in the management of poisoning with methanol and ethylene glycol which are also metabolised by alcohol and aldehyde dehydrogenases.

MECHANISMS OF TOXICITY
- Ethanol initially disinhibits the brain and behaviour.

- Subsequent doses depress the brain, including respiration and blood pressure and body temperature control.

- Ethanol potentiates the CNS depressant effects of other psychotropic drugs.

- Ethanol has a direct irritant effect on the gastric mucosa.

CLINICAL FEATURES

Clinical features of poisoning with ethanol	
Early	**Late**
Enhanced well-being	Nausea
Increased talkativeness	Vomiting
Increased extroversion	Increasing drowsiness
Dizziness	Coma
Nystagmus	Hypotension
Ataxia	Hypothermia
Dysarthria	Respiratory depression
	Inhalation of gastric contents

LABORATORY FEATURES
- Ethanol is the commonest reason for an increased plasma osmolality.

- Hypoglycaemia is an uncommon complication most likely to be encountered in children.

- There may be a mild metabolic acidosis.

- Fluoride oxalate should be used as anticoagulant.

- Blood ethanol concentrations over 8 g/L have been recorded in survivors.

- Different units of concentration g/L, mg%, mmol/L are in use, the base unit should be the litre.

- Typically fatalities are associated with ethanol concentrations greater than 4 g/L.

MANAGEMENT
- Management is supportive with attention to the airway, adequacy of ventilation, and correction of hypotension and hypothermia.

- Hypoglycaemia should be corrected if detected.

- The acidosis is unlikely to be of such severity as to require correction.

- Dialysis (preferably haemodialysis) readily eliminates ethanol but is highly unlikely ever to be indicated, even in patients with severe CNS depression and high blood alcohol concentrations.

ETHYLENE GLYCOL

IMPORTANT FACTS
- Ethylene glycol poisoning is uncommon, but is frequently severe and fatal.

- Diagnosis requires a high index of suspicion.

- Ethylene glycol is a component of antifreezes and vehicle windscreen washes (often in association with methanol).

- Early intervention is required to minimise morbidity and mortality.

- Mortality increases with increasing acidosis.

- Alcohol dehydrogenase has a much higher affinity for ethanol than for ethylene glycol.

- Fomepizole (4-methylpyrazole) is now available to inhibit alcohol dehydrogenase and appears to be preferable to treatment with ethanol.

MECHANISMS OF TOXICITY
- Ethylene glycol depresses the central nervous system, but is relatively non-toxic in itself.

- Toxicity results from metabolic activation to glycolaldehyde then to glycolic acid (the main metabolite), and glyoxylic and oxalic acids by alcohol and aldehyde dehydrogenases respectively.

CLINICAL FEATURES

Clinical features of poisoning with ethylene glycol	
Common	**Uncommon**
Nausea	Convulsions
Vomiting	Cranial nerve abnormalities
Ataxia	Cardiac arrhythmias
Dysarthria	Cardiac failure
Drowsiness	Myositis
	Renal failure
	Cerebral oedema

The onset of features is commonly delayed, particularly when ethanol is ingested along with the ethylene glycol.

LABORATORY FEATURES

- Severe metabolic acidosis with a high anion gap is an important diagnostic and prognostic feature.

- A high osmolar gap may also be present.

- Urine obtained within a few hours of ingestion may fluoresce under an ultraviolet lamp if an antifreeze has been ingested – some contain fluorescein.

- Oxalate crystals may be present in the urine.

- Hypocalcaemia may be severe as calcium combines with oxalic acid to precipitate in tissues as calcium oxalate.

- Creatine kinase activity may be increased if myositis develops.

PLASMA CONCENTRATIONS

- Optimum management requires urgent measurement of plasma ethylene glycol concentrations – treatment must not be delayed until acidosis indicates the development of severe toxicity.

- Plasma ethanol concentrations may also need to be measured to monitor treatment, especially if haemodialysis is used.

MANAGEMENT

- Gastric lavage for patients who present within one hour of ingestion of a substantial amount.

- Activated charcoal is of no value – it does not adsorb ethylene glycol.

- Measure the plasma ethylene glycol concentration.

- Give ethanol (by mouth if the patient is conscious – otherwise by intravenous infusion) to slow the rate of metabolism of ethylene glycol; alcohol dehydrogenase has a significantly greater affinity for ethanol than for ethylene glycol.

- Correct acidosis as required – large amounts of sodium bicarbonate may have to be infused with the concomitant risk of hypernatraemia.

- Correct hypocalcaemia as required.

- Haemodialysis is the elimination technique of choice in clinically severe poisoning indicated by severe metabolic acidosis and plasma ethylene glycol concentrations exceeding 500 mg/L. Rebound rises can occur on cessation of haemodialysis.

- Haemodialysis should be continued until ethylene glycol can no longer be detected in the plasma.

- Fomepizole may obviate the need for ethanol treatment, haemodialysis and monitoring of ethylene glycol concentrations, but is currently expensive and not widely available.

HYDROGEN FLUORIDE AND FLUORIDE SALTS

IMPORTANT FACTS
- Fluoride poisoning may result from ingestion, inhalation or skin exposure.

- Hydrogen fluoride (hydrofluoric acid) poisoning is rare and usually encountered in an industrial setting; skin, eye and occasionally inhalation are the usual routes of exposure.

- The most common scenario of fluoride overdose in clinical practice is that of young children accidentally ingesting sodium fluoride tablets prescribed for dental caries prophylaxis although this rarely results in serious consequences.

MECHANISMS OF TOXICITY
- Hydrogen fluoride is a potent corrosive agent.

- Fluoride ions chelate calcium causing hypocalcaemia.

- Fluoride inhibits glycolytic enzymes, cholinesterases and magnesium and manganese metal enzymes.

- Fluoride is neurotoxic and myotoxic.

CLINICAL FEATURES – SYSTEMIC TOXICITY
Absorption of fluoride by any route may result in:
- muscle weakness
- paraesthesiae
- tetany
- convulsions
- hypotension
- cardiac arrhythmias (including ventricular fibrillation) secondary to hypocalcaemia.

CLINICAL FEATURES – DIRECT TOXICITY
SKIN CONTACT
- Immediate pain from contamination by concentrated solutions.

- Pain may not occur with dilute solutions but skin and systemic toxicity may still develop if contact is prolonged.

- Coagulative necrosis of the skin.

- Skin ulcers that are often painful and slow to heal.

EYE CONTACT
- Pain in the eye.

- Tear production.

- Blepharospasm.

- Corneal ulceration.

INHALATION (HYDROGEN FLUORIDE)
- Choking.

- Cough.

- Breathlessness.

- Cyanosis.

- Laryngeal oedema.

- Pulmonary oedema.

INGESTION
- Ingestion of dental caries prophylaxis tablets rarely causes serious toxicity.

- Rapid onset of nausea.

- Vomiting.

- Abdominal pain.

- Diarrhoea.

- Corrosive injury to the mouth, oesophagus, stomach and possibly larynx with hydrofluoric acid only.

- Systemic features secondary to hypocalcaemia (see above).

- Coma.

- Liver and renal failure.

LABORATORY FEATURES
- Hypocalcaemia and hypomagnesaemia are frequently severe.

- Coagulation abnormalities secondary to hypocalcaemia.

PLASMA CONCENTRATIONS
- Are of no value in the management of poisoning.

MANAGEMENT

ALL CASES
- A clear airway and adequate ventilation should be ensured as necessary.

- Hypocalcaemia must be corrected with intravenous calcium gluconate (10%).

- Hypomagnesaemia must also be corrected with with Mg SO_4 (20 mmol/day i.v. for an adult).

- Cardiac arrhythmias should be managed conventionally.

SKIN CONTACT
- Wash contaminated skin with copious quantities of water for at least 15 minutes, even in the absence of pain or obvious burns.

- Immerse painful burns in ice-cold water until the pain subsides.

- Coat burns repeatedly with 2.5% calcium gluconate gel.

- Injection of 10% calcium gluconate solution around burns may relieve persistent pain.

EYE CONTACT
- Irrigate the conjunctival sac with water or normal (0.9%) saline for at least 15 minutes.

- Instillation of local anaesthetic solutions may be necessary to achieve satisfactory irrigation.

- Refer for ophthalmological assessment.

INHALATION

- The casualty will have been removed from the toxic atmosphere by the emergency services.

- Give oxygen.

- Mechanical ventilation may be required for pulmonary oedema.

INGESTION

- Gastric lavage is contraindicated if hydrofluoric acid has been ingested.

- Activated charcoal is of no value.

- Give milk or, if available, soluble calcium tablets (10 – 20 g) if a fluoride salt has been ingested. This will chelate fluoride remaining in the gut.

HYPOGLYCAEMIC DRUGS

IMPORTANT FACTS

- Intentional insulin overdose is uncommon.

- Intentional overdoses of oral hypoglycaemic agents are less common still.

- Overdose is most likely to occur in diabetics, their close relatives and healthcare professionals.

- Occasionally, hypoglycaemia induced by drugs is encountered in Munchausen's syndrome or Munchausen's syndrome by proxy. Hypoglycaemia due to this cause is commonly referred to as factitious.

- Unexplained hypoglycaemia found on routine screening may be the only clue to the diagnosis; drug-induced hypoglycaemia is much more likely than hypoglycaemia secondary to an insulinoma.

- Despite the massive doses of insulin commonly injected in overdose, hypoglycaemia may not be severe.

- Overdose with both insulin and oral hypoglycaemic agents (particularly chlorpropamide which has a long half-life) is likely to cause prolonged hypoglycaemia.

MECHANISMS OF TOXICITY

- Insulin lowers plasma glucose concentrations by driving glucose from the extracellular compartment into tissues.

- Overdosage of oral hypoglycaemic drugs stimulates the pancreas to release insulin, leading to high circulating insulin activity.

- Insulin receptor down-regulation may account for the fact that insulin-induced hypoglycaemia is sometimes not as severe as might be expected.

CLINICAL FEATURES

Clinical features of poisoning with hypoglycaemic agents	
Common	**Uncommon**
Drowsiness	Cerebral infarction and oedema
Sweating	Peripheral circulatory failure
Coma	Pulmonary oedema
Convulsions	Metabolic acidosis
Hyporeflexia	
Extensor plantar responses	
Hyperventilation	
Sinus tachycardia	

LABORATORY FEATURES

- Hypoglycaemia.

- Hypokalaemia.

PLASMA CONCENTRATIONS

- Concentrations of oral hypoglycaemic agents are of no value in the management of poisoning.

- Plasma insulin concentrations may be greatly elevated and remain so for 3-4 days after overdoses of both insulin and oral agents.

MANAGEMENT

- Blood should be taken for the emergency measurement of the glucose concentration.

- If covert insulin administration is suspected take blood, preferably while the patient is hypoglycaemic, for measurement of insulin and C-peptide concentrations; high insulin concentrations in the absence of C-peptide confirm the suspicion.

- Hypoglycaemia demands the administration of intravenous glucose (50 mL of 50%) irrespective of ingestion of an oral hypoglycaemic drug.

- Start a constant infusion of glucose (19-20%) into a large (preferably central) vein.

- Glucagon is unlikely to be effective.

- Once the patient is stabilised, gastric lavage should be considered for patients who present within one hour of ingestion of a substantial overdose of an oral hypoglycaemic agent.

- Monitor plasma glucose concentrations – recurrent hypoglycaemia is common.

- Encourage the patient to consume carbohydrate-rich meals once they are able to eat.

- Intravenous diazoxide may be the best approach to treating overdoses of oral hypoglycaemic drugs – in contrast to glucose, it blocks insulin release while increasing blood glucose. Octreotide is a possible alternative to diazoxide.

IRON SALTS

IMPORTANT FACTS
- Serious iron poisoning is uncommon, but may be fatal in adults as well as children.

- Numerous products containing iron salts, frequently co-formulated with vitamins are available without prescription.

- The toxicity of an iron-containing preparation depends on its elemental iron content and not on its weight of salt. The amount taken in overdose is rarely known with certainty. The following dose/toxicity relationships have been proposed:

Dose/toxicity relationships in poisoning with iron salts	
Dose of elemental iron mg/kg	Toxicity
<20	no/mild
>20	moderate
>150	serious/death

These correlations should be viewed as general statements; what happens in practice is more important.

- Absorption of iron from the gut is poor.

- The kinetics of iron after acute overdose have not been adequately studied – the available evidence suggests that plasma concentrations peak early (within 3-4 h) and decline rapidly. Interpretation of a single concentration without consideration of time since ingestion is, therefore, inherently suspect.

- There is no single measure of the severity of poisoning.

MECHANISMS OF TOXICITY
- Direct irritation, staining and ulceration of the pyloric antrum and upper small bowel.

- Impairment of mitochondrial function, particularly in periportal hepatocytes, leading to necrosis.

- Hypotension and reduced cardiac output secondary to direct effects on arterioles and the myocardium or release of vaso-active substances.

CLINICAL FEATURES
- The course of acute iron intoxication has been divided into phases but these are of doubtful value.

- Direct irritation of the gastrointestinal tract is the cause of the common features of poisoning.

- Systemic toxicity occurs when plasma iron concentrations exceed total iron binding capacity.

- Very few patients develop systemic toxicity.

- Potentially lethal poisoning is characterised by the presence of uncommon features that indicate systemic toxicity secondary to absorption of significant quantities of iron.

- Unless a plain abdominal x-ray is taken within two hours it may be misleading due to tablet dissolution.

Clinical features of poisoning with iron salts	
Common (direct toxicity)	**Uncommon (systemic toxicity)**
Nausea	Shock
Vomiting (grey or black coloured)	GI haemorrhage
Abdominal pain	Impaired consciousness
Grey/black diarrhoea	Hepatic necrosis and its complications
Acidosis	Acute renal failure

LABORATORY FEATURES
- Polymorph leucocytosis.

- Hyperglycaemia may be present in the early stages.

- Acidosis – if present early, is probably the single most important laboratory indicator of serious poisoning.

- Increased ALT/AST activities if liver damage occurs.

- Hypoglycaemia, prothrombin time prolongation or raised INR and other features of hepatic necrosis.

- After treatment with desferrioxamine the urine may turn red (*vin rosé*) due to the presence of ferrioxamine, the desferrioxamine/iron chelate.

- Minor prolongation of the INR may be present early in the course of acute iron poisoning due to interference with the assay. Prolongation at a later stage reflects hypoprothrombinaemia secondary to acute hepatic necrosis.

PLASMA IRON CONCENTRATIONS

- Plasma iron concentrations are commonly within normal limits – grossly elevated concentrations are rare. Concentrations of <55, 55-90 and >90 µmol/L approximately four hours post-ingestion have been said to correlate with mild, moderate and severe toxicity respectively but the validity of the claim is unproven. Samples should be taken 4 hours or more post-ingestion. Samples must not be haemolysed.

- Colourimetric iron assays are unreliable in the presence of desferrioxamine.

- The plasma iron binding capacity may be falsely raised and therefore, should not be measured.

MANAGEMENT

IMMEDIATE – ALL CASES

- Gastric lavage for patients who present within one hour of ingestion of a substantial overdose.

- Activated charcoal is of no value – it does not adsorb iron salts.

PATIENTS WITH SYSTEMIC TOXICITY

- Give desferrioxamine immediately – do not wait for the result of the plasma iron concentration.

PATIENTS WITHOUT EVIDENCE OF SYSTEMIC TOXICITY

- Measure the plasma iron concentration.

- Do not measure the plasma iron binding capacity.

- Give desferrioxamine if the plasma iron concentration exceeds the anticipated total iron binding capacity – this usually means concentrations in excess of 90 μmol/L (5 mg/L).

SUPPORTIVE CARE
- Monitor liver and renal function.

- Monitor blood glucose and correct hypoglycaemia as required.

- Correct acidosis as required.

- Manage hepatic and renal failure conventionally.

LEAD

IMPORTANT FACTS

- Lead exposure in adults is commonly chronic and occupational in origin, particularly in the scrap metal industry and manufacture of batteries and ceramics.

- Children may ingest lead by chewing on surfaces painted with lead-containing pigments or eating contaminated soil.

- Ingestion of, and poisoning by, lead has also been reported after the use of ceramic vessels and cosmetics ('surma') containing lead-based powders.

- Poisoning may also result from inhalation or dermal absorption of tetraethyl lead found in leaded petrol.

- Lead is readily absorbed by inhalation but only some 10-15% of that ingested is absorbed.

- 95% of absorbed lead is deposited in the bones and teeth.

- Virtually all of the lead in the blood is in the red blood cells.

- Endogenous elimination of lead is extremely slow.

MECHANISM OF TOXICITY

- Lead variably inhibits the enzymes involved in the synthesis of haem.

CLINICAL FEATURES

Clinical features of lead poisoning	
Common	**Uncommon**
Lethargy	Vomiting
Abdominal discomfort	Abdominal pain
	Constipation
	Encephalopathy (seizures, mania, delirium, coma)
	Lead lines on the gums (bluish discolouration of the margins caused by deposition of lead sulphide)
	Motor peripheral neuropathy leading to foot and wrist drop

LABORATORY FEATURES
- Glycosuria, aminoaciduria and phosphaturia secondary to renal tubular dysfunction (reversible).

- Renal impairment secondary to renal interstitial fibrosis (irreversible).

- Red cell life span is decreased.

- Microcytic or normocytic, hypochromic anaemia.

- Red cells may show punctate basophilia.

- Haemolytic anaemia may complicate severe poisoning.

- Increased amounts of ∂-aminolaevulinic acid are found in blood and urine.

- Free erythrocyte protoporphyrin concentrations are increased.

- Urinary coproporphyrin and free erythrocyte protoporphyrin concentrations may also be increased.

- Erythrocyte zinc protoporphyrin concentrations are also increased.

BLOOD CONCENTRATIONS
- Blood lead concentrations exceeding 3.4 µmol/L (700 µg/L) require workers to be removed from further immediate exposure.

- Blood lead concentrations exceeding 0.49 µmol/L (100 µg/L) have been associated with illness in children.

- A urine lead concentration exceeding 0.73 µmol/L (150 µg/L) indicates excess exposure in those working with organic lead compounds.

MANAGEMENT
- Identification of the source of the lead and prevention of further exposure is an immediate priority.

- The blood lead concentration should be measured and, if possible, the total body lead burden estimated by X-ray fluorescence.

- A combination of symptoms, blood lead concentrations and total body lead burden is used to decide those patients who should be treated with chelating agents.

- The chelating agent of choice depends on the severity of poisoning and whether the person is an in-patient or an out-patient. Sodium calcium edetate is effective in acute and chronic lead intoxication, but has to be given intravenously. Dimercaptosuccinic acid (DMSA) is a less efficient chelator on a molar basis, but has the advantage that it can be given orally.

LITHIUM

IMPORTANT FACTS
- Many therapeutic lithium formulations on the UK market are of a modified release type.

- There are three common clinical scenarios; therapeutic overdosage, acute over dosage superimposed on therapeutic doses and acute overdose in patients not on long-term treatment.

- Life-threatening toxicity is more commonly the result of therapeutic excess rather than acute massive overdose.

MECHANISMS OF TOXICITY
- The mechanism of action of lithium is not known.

- The concentration in neurones determines the presence or otherwise of toxicity.

- Lithium appears to distribute only slowly from the extracellular fluid into cells.

CLINICAL FEATURES
The onset of features of toxicity may be delayed for up to 12 hours or even longer. In general, acute overdose or acute overdose superimposed on long-term therapy seldom causes toxicity.

Clinical features of poisoning with lithium	
Common	**Uncommon**
Nausea	Nephrogenic diabetes insipidus
Vomiting	Renal failure
Diarrhoea	Coma
Drowsiness	Convulsions
Tremor	Polyneuropathy
Increased muscle tone	
Rigidity	
Fasciculation	
Myoclonus	

LABORATORY FEATURES
- Hypernatraemia may be secondary to nephrogenic diabetes insipidus and/or exacerbated by saline infusions.

- Evidence of impaired renal function.

SERUM CONCENTRATIONS
- Serum is the preferred sample type to ensure samples are not collected in lithium heparin tubes.

- Serum lithium concentrations correlate poorly with clinical features because of the slow distribution across cell membranes.

- Concentrations should be measured 6 hours post ingestion.

- Acute overdose and acute overdose superimposed on long-term therapy are commonly associated with plasma concentrations well above the therapeutic range but with no toxicity.

- Therapeutic intoxication may occur with only mildly elevated plasma concentrations.

- Clinical recovery from lithium poisoning lags many hours behind reduction in plasma concentrations.

- Haemodialysis should be considered when plasma lithium concentrations exceeding 7.5 mmol/L in acute overdose and 4.0 mmol/L in acute on chronic or therapeutic overdose respectively are associated with neurological features and impaired renal function.

MANAGEMENT
- Gastric lavage for patients who present within one hour of ingestion of a substantial overdose.

- Activated charcoal is of no value – it does not adsorb lithium.

- Monitor serum lithium concentrations.

- Forced diuresis is of no value.

- Haemodialysis is the treatment of choice for poisoning with neurological features, rebound rises may occur up to 6 hours post haemodialysis due to redistribution of lithium from cells to the extracellular fluid.

- Caution when infusing saline; hypernatraemia is a hazard.

MERCURY

IMPORTANT FACTS

- Metallic mercury is volatile at room temperature.

- Metallic mercury is poorly absorbed from the gut but mercury vapour is well absorbed through the lungs.

- Volatility increases as environmental temperature rises – potentially toxic inhalation concentrations may be attained in confined spaces.

- Mercury poisoning is primarily occupational in origin.

- Non-occupational mercury is obtained from food (particularly fish) and dental amalgam.

- In practice, metallic mercury exposure is most commonly the result of ingestion of the broken bulbs of clinical thermometers.

- Young children commonly accidentally swallow button batteries containing mercuric oxide – potentially toxic blood mercury concentrations may be attained if the battery disintegrates during its passage through the gut.

- Rarely, individuals with ready access to metallic mercury (often dental technicians) inject themselves with it.

- Mercurous mercury compounds are largely non-toxic.

- Fungicidal seed dressings were formerly an important source of organomercury compounds if the treated grain was used for food rather than planting; they are no longer used.

- The kidneys are the main storage depot for inorganic mercury and the brain for organic mercury.

MECHANISMS OF TOXICITY

- Mercury attaches itself to sulphydryl groups and inhibits a variety of enzymes.

- Mercuric mercury compounds are corrosive (mercuric chloride is known as corrosive sublimate).

CLINICAL FEATURES

ACUTE POISONING – INHALATION OF MERCURY VAPOUR

Clinical features of acute poisoning – inhalation of mercury vapour	
Common	**Uncommon**
Cough	Pneumonitis
Chest tightness	Pulmonary oedema
Retrosternal discomfort	Nephrotic syndrome
Bronchiolitis	Tremor
	Neuropsychiatric features
	Peripheral neuropathy

INGESTION

- Metallic mercury does not cause toxic features.

- Mercuric chloride and other inorganic mercuric salts cause abdominal colic, blood-stained diarrhoea, ulceration of the gastrointestinal mucosa and shock.

- Mercurous chloride (calomel) induces diarrhoea but, like other mercurous compounds, it is absorbed less well and is correspondingly less toxic than mercuric salts.

INTRAVENOUS OR SUBCUTANEOUS INJECTION OF METALLIC MERCURY

- Pulmonary or soft-tissue foreign body reaction with granuloma formation in the long term.

CHRONIC POISONING

Clinical features of chronic mercury poisoning	
Inorganic mercury compounds	**Organomercury compounds**
Anorexia	Paraesthesiae of the lips and extremities
Insomnia	Unsteadiness
Sweating	Ataxia
Increased excitability	Tremor
Tremor	Dysarthria
Gingivitis	Visual field constriction
Hypersalivation	Emotional lability
Emotional lability	
Impaired memory	
Renal tubular damage and acidosis	

LABORATORY FEATURES
- Proteinuria.

- Aminoaciduria.

- Features of renal tubular acidosis.

BLOOD CONCENTRATIONS
- Blood concentrations of 500 nmol/L (100 µg/L) in patients with symptoms or values greater than 1000 nmol/L (200 µg/L) require chelation therapy.

URINE MERCURY/CREATININE RATIOS
Urine mercury/creatinine ratios are used as a measure of exposure to mercury. The significance of values is given below:

The significance of urine mercury/creatinine ratios	
Urine mercury/creatinine ratio nmol/mmol	**Significance**
<5.5	Normal
<40	Acceptable
40-100	Monitor and investigate
>100	Remove from exposure

MANAGEMENT

ACUTE SYSTEMIC TOXICITY
- Give dimercaprol (British Anti-Lewisite, BAL) for inorganic mercury poisoning.

- Give oral DMPS (unithiol) or DMSA (succimer) to enhance mercury elimination, protect against renal damage, and increase survival. DMPS improves neurological features and may be more effective than DMSA.

- Give either DMSA or DMPS for methyl mercury poisoning.

ACUTE INHALATION
- The victim must be removed from the toxic atmosphere.

- The inspired oxygen concentration should be increased.

- Mechanical ventilation may be required for pulmonary oedema.

- The role of corticosteroids is not clear.

ACUTE INGESTION
- Gastric emptying is contraindicated when mercuric salts have been ingested.

- Swallowed metallic mercury does not require treatment.

- Button batteries releasing mercuric oxide should be removed surgically.

INJECTION
- Mercury injected intravenously or intra-arterially is clearly beyond retrieval.

- Surgically drain subcutaneous metallic mercury if the collection is sufficiently well circumscribed.

CHRONIC SYSTEMIC TOXICITY
- There is no effective treatment for chronic mercury poisoning.

METHANOL

IMPORTANT FACTS

- Methanol poisoning is uncommon but is frequently severe and fatal. Diagnosis requires a high index of suspicion.

- Methanol is a component of antifreezes and vehicle windscreen washes (often in association with ethylene glycol) and is sometimes used as a fuel.

- Early intervention is required to minimise morbidity and mortality.

- Alcohol dehydrogenase has a much higher affinity for ethanol than for methanol.

- Fomepizole (4-methylpyrazole) is now available to inhibit alcohol dehydrogenase and appears to be preferable to treatment with ethanol.

MECHANISMS OF TOXICITY

- Methanol is relatively non-toxic before metabolism; it causes minor central nervous system depression.

- The major toxicity results from metabolic activation to formaldehyde then rapidly to formic acid by alcohol and aldehyde dehydrogenases respectively. Formic acid is considered to be the major cause of acidosis.

- Lactate production may contribute to the acidosis in the later stages of poisoning.

CLINICAL FEATURES

Clinical features of methanol poisoning	
Common	**Uncommon**
Nausea	Blindness
Vomiting	Convulsions
Abdominal pain	Kussmaul's respiration
Headache	Pancreatitis
Blurred vision	Respiratory failure
Breathlessness	Hypotension
Sweating	Cerebral oedema
Restlessness	Basal ganglia infarction

The onset of features is commonly delayed, particularly when ethanol is ingested along with methanol.

LABORATORY FEATURES
- Severe metabolic acidosis with a high anion gap is the only important feature.

- A high osmolal gap may also be present.

- Urine obtained within a few hours of ingestion may fluoresce under an ultraviolet lamp if an antifreeze has been ingested – some contain fluorescein.

PLASMA CONCENTRATIONS
- Optimum management requires urgent measurement of plasma methanol concentrations – treatment must not be delayed until acidosis indicates the development of severe toxicity as delay may allow serious neurological and ocular morbidity.

- Plasma ethanol concentrations may also need to be measured to monitor treatment, especially if haemodialysis is used.

MANAGEMENT
- Gastric lavage for patients who present within one hour of ingestion of a substantial overdose.

- Activated charcoal is of no value – it does not adsorb methanol.

- Measure the plasma methanol concentration.

- Give ethanol (by mouth if the patient is conscious – otherwise by intravenous infusion) to slow the rate of metabolism of methanol.

- Correct acidosis as required – large amounts of sodium bicarbonate may have to be infused, with hypernatraemia as a concomitant hazard.

- Haemodialysis is the elimination technique of choice in patients with clouded mental function, severe metabolic acidosis and plasma methanol concentrations exceeding 500 mg/L. Haemodialysis should be continued until the plasma methanol concentration is less than 50 mg/L.

- Fomepizole, while not yet licensed for methanol poisoning may obviate the need for ethanol treatment, haemodialysis and monitoring of methanol concentrations, but is currently expensive and not widely available.

OPIATE AND OPIOID ANALGESICS

IMPORTANT FACTS
- The opiate and opioid analgesics commonly encountered in clinical practice include dextropropoxyphene, codeine, dihydrocodeine, heroin (diamorphine or diacetyl-morphine), morphine, methadone and buprenorphine.

- Dihydrocodeine, heroin, morphine, methadone and buprenorphine overdose is almost completely confined to individuals who are dependent on such drugs.

- Poisoning with the most potent opiates and opioids may result from injection and inhalation as well as ingestion.

- Co-proxamol contains enough dextropropoxyphene to cause life-threatening opioid toxicity, particularly when an overdose is taken with ethanol.

- Overdoses of codeine co-formulated with paracetamol or aspirin seldom lead to opioid toxicity.

- Hepatitis B and HIV infection are important risks in injecting users.

MECHANISMS OF TOXICITY
- Opiate/opioid analgesics are potent CNS and respiratory depressants.

- They may also have an effect on the alveolo-capillary membrane of the lungs rendering it more permeable.

CLINICAL FEATURES

Clinical features of poisoning with opiate and opioid analgesics	
Common	**Uncommon**
Nausea	Convulsions
Vomiting	Skin blisters
Drowsiness progressing to coma	Rhabdomyolysis
A very low respiratory rate	Hypotension
Pin-point pupils	Peripheral circulatory failure
	Cardiac conduction defects and arrhythmias
	Hypothermia
	Pulmonary oedema
	Renal failure

LABORATORY FEATURES

- Hypoxaemia.

- Hypercapnia in severe cases.

- Increased serum creatine kinase activity if skeletal muscle has been damaged.

PLASMA CONCENTRATIONS

- Are of no value in the management of poisoning.

MANAGEMENT

EMERGENCY MEASURES

- Establish a clear airway.

- Assist ventilation if necessary.

- Give oxygen.

- Give naloxone intravenously as soon as possible.

- Once the patient has been stabilised, consider gastric lavage for those who have ingested the overdose and present within one hour.

REVERSAL OF OPIATE/OPIOID EFFECTS

Naloxone (0.8-1.2 mg as an intravenous bolus in an adult) can be expected to produce dramatic clinical improvement. Within 1-2 minutes there should be:

- a dramatic return to consciousness,
- an increase in the respiratory rate,
- a considerable increase in the size of the pupils.

If there is no response, or an incomplete response, to naloxone, consider:

- is the diagnosis of opiate/opioid overdose robust?

- was the dose of naloxone adequate? Naloxone is a competitive antagonist and the greater the concentration of opiate/opioid at receptor sites, the greater the amount of antagonist required to reverse intoxication. Repeat naloxone every 1-2 minutes to a total of at least 5 mg.

- could the opioid be buprenorphine? – its effects cannot be reversed by even large doses of naloxone,

- could the opioid be pentazocine? – very large doses of naloxone may be necessary,

- has the patient taken other CNS depressants as well?

- could there have been hypoxic brain damage before reaching medical care?

MAINTAINING REVERSAL OF OPIATE/OPIOID EFFECTS

Naloxone has a very short half-life (30-60 minutes). Repeated doses are therefore often required to maintain reversal of opiate/opioid intoxication when:

- poisoning is severe (suggesting high concentrations of the toxin at receptor sites),

- methadone, an opioid with a particularly long half-life, is involved.

Careful clinical observation with repeated bolus doses of naloxone being given if signs of toxicity return is essential in such circumstances. A constant intravenous infusion of naloxone can be used but this approach does not diminish the importance of intensive observation and bolus doses of antagonist as clinically indicated.

MANAGEMENT OF COMPLICATIONS

- Convulsions are not suppressed by naloxone. Correct hypoxia and acidosis and give intravenous diazepam if necessary.

- Cardiac arrhythmias are not suppressed by naloxone. Correct hypoxia and acidosis and manage conventionally.

- Give high-flow oxygen for acute pulmonary oedema. Mechanical ventilation may be required.

- Peripheral circulatory failure and oliguria may respond to inotropes.

- Skin blisters are managed as burns.

- Rhabdomyolysis is managed conventionally.

ORGANOPHOSPHATE INSECTICIDES

IMPORTANT FACTS

- Organophosphates are readily absorbed through the gut, respiratory tract and skin.

- Organophosphate (OP) insecticides are alleged to be the cause of thousands of deaths and non-fatal poisonings annually in the third world.

- In developed societies public concern is centred on possible long-term ill-health from single or repeated exposures to low concentrations of OPs.

- Not all OPs are cholinesterase inhibitors.

MECHANISMS OF TOXICITY

- OP insecticides and military nerve gases inhibit acetylcholinesterase.

- The speed of onset, severity and duration of toxicity caused by individual organophosphates vary considerably and depend on a number of factors.

- High tissue concentrations of insecticide and high affinity of the enzyme for it, increase toxicity.

- The faster the insecticide-enzyme complex hydrolyses (thus 'reactivating' the enzyme), the less is the intensity and the shorter is the duration of poisoning.

- The OP-enzyme complex undergoes 'ageing', a chemical change thought to be mono-dealkylation, that prevents both spontaneous and oxime-induced reactivation.

- Once the OP-cholinesterase complex has aged recovery depends on the synthesis of new acetylcholinesterase.

CLINICAL FEATURES

ACUTE POISONING

It is customary to classify the features of poisoning by cholinesterase inhibitors into muscarinic and nicotinic. The latter occur mainly at neuromuscular junctions. Muscarinic features usually occur first and in the alimentary or respiratory tract depending on which is the route of exposure.

Clinical features of acute poisoning with organophosphate insecticides	
Muscarinic	**Nicotinic**
Anxiety	Fasciculation
Restlessness	Increasing muscle flaccidity
Dizziness	Muscle weakness
Salivation	(including the external eye muscles and the
Tear production	muscles of respiration)
Bronchorrhoea	
Bronchospasm	
Abdominal colic	
Urgency of micturition	
Urgent bowel movements	
Sinus bradycardia	

Tachycardia occurs but not as frequently as one might expect from the mode of action of these compounds. Respiratory failure is the usual cause of death and results from a combination of depressed respiratory drive, reduced ventilation secondary to weakness of the respiratory muscles and airways obstruction caused by bronchospasm and retention of bronchial secretions. Severe poisoning may also be complicated by convulsions, coma and cardiac arrhythmias.

LABORATORY FEATURES
• Red cell cholinesterase (acetylcholinesterase) and serum cholinesterase (pseudo-cholinesterase or butyryl cholinesterase) activities are both reduced.

• Hyperglycaemia and glycosuria are common.

CHOLINESTERASE ACTIVITY
A diagnosis of OP poisoning can be confirmed by demonstrating reduced serum or, preferably, erythrocyte cholinesterase activity. Cholinesterase activity is commonly in the range:

   • 50-70% of normal in asymptomatic patients.
   • 10-20% in moderate poisoning.
   • less than 10% in severe poisoning.

LONG-TERM HEALTH EFFECTS
Organophosphates in sheep dips are alleged to be responsible for long-term debilitating illness with symptoms such as:

- lethargy,
- irritability,
- inability to concentrate,
- depression,
- variable mood,
- disturbed sleep,
- paraesthesiae,
- muscle aches.

In some cases the symptoms are so severe that the individual is greatly disabled, housebound and with a poor quality of life. Clinical examination and laboratory tests usually fail to detect abnormalities. Subtle impairment of nerve conduction velocities and performance in some neurobehavioural tests have been reported but their relevance to the symptoms is unclear.

MANAGEMENT

SUPPORTIVE TREATMENT
- Ensure a clear airway and adequate ventilation.

- Remove bronchial secretions as often as necessary.

- Give high inspired oxygen concentration.

- Control convulsions with intravenous diazepam.

- Even in the absence of convulsions, diazepam, 5-10 mg intravenously for an adult, reduces anxiety and restlessness and may improve the outcome.

- Once the patient's condition is stabilised, consider gastric lavage if a substantial amount has been ingested within the previous hour.

ANTIDOTES
- Atropine blocks the muscarinic effects of organophosphates. It is given intravenously and repeated at 10-30 minute intervals until bronchorrhoea and bronchospasm are abolished or there is evidence of atropine intoxication (i.e. dry mouth, tachycardia, dry skin, vasodilatation).

- Large doses of atropine (30 mg or more in the first 24 hours) may be necessary in adults who are severely poisoned.

- Smaller amounts of atropine may be sufficient if oximes such as pralidoxime are also given.

- Pralidoxime mesylate (P$_2$S, PAMM) in a dose of 30 mg/kg body weight by slow intravenous injection reactivates phosphorylated cholinesterase and should preferably be given before ageing of the enzyme-OP complex occurs. Clinical improvement can be expected within about 30 minutes and is evidenced by reduction of the nicotinic effects and convulsions, and improvement in conscious level.

- Give further doses of pralidoxime at 4 hour intervals if features of poisoning persist and for as long as red cell and plasma cholinesterase activities are reduced.

- Pralidoxime may still be of benefit relatively late in the course of poisoning.

PARACETAMOL (ACETAMINOPHEN)

IMPORTANT FACTS
- Paracetamol (acetaminophen) is the single most important substance involved in childhood and adult poisonings in the UK.

- Paracetamol overdose is the most important cause of fulminant hepatic failure in the UK.

- Only a small minority of overdoses develop hepatic failure.

- Children are at less risk of paracetamol-induced liver damage than adults.

MECHANISMS OF TOXICITY
- N-acetyl-p-benzoquinoneimine (NAPQI), a minor metabolite of therapeutic doses of paracetamol, is produced in potentially toxic amounts after overdose.

- NAPQI is rendered harmless by conjugation with glutathione.

- After paracetamol overdose hepatic glutathione stores may be rapidly depleted leaving NAPQI to bind to cell proteins and cause cell death.

- Substances that induce microsomal oxidases (anticonvulsants, ethanol, rifampicin) are widely believed to predispose to paracetamol-induced hepatic necrosis by increasing the rate at which NAPQI is formed.

- Anorexia nervosa and AIDS are also widely believed to predispose to hepatic necrosis by virtue of reducing the amount of hepatic glutathione available to bind NAPQI.

CLINICAL FEATURES
- Vomiting, due to the drug, may be the only feature in the first 12 hours after ingestion.

- Later vomiting (12-36 hours after overdose) is likely to be due to the onset of liver necrosis.

- Right upper quadrant abdominal pain 24 hours or more after overdose is due to hepatic damage and swelling and stretching of the liver capsule.

- Jaundice may become clinically apparent 36-72 hours after ingestion.

- Hypoglycaemia may complicate severe liver damage.

- Peak abnormalities of liver function tests occur 72-96 hours after the overdose.

- Hepatic encephalopathy may develop from about 72 hours onwards.

- Cerebral oedema and brain stem coning may complicate hepatic encephalopathy from about 96 hours onwards.

- Acute renal failure complicates about 15% of cases of severe liver damage.

UNCOMMON CLINICAL FEATURES
- Rarely, acute renal failure may develop in the absence of severe liver damage.

- Coma with metabolic acidosis and grossly high plasma paracetamol concentrations.

LABORATORY FEATURES
- Dipstick haematuria about 24 hours or more after overdose may indicate renal tubular damage.

- Paracetamol metabolites may make the urine brownish in colour.

- Patients with early (within 24 hours) acidosis are likely to develop severe liver damage.

- Severe liver damage is defined as an ALT or AST activity exceeding 1000 IU/L.

- Peak ALT or AST abnormalities occur at about 96 hours after the overdose.

- Peak ALT or AST activities of 15000 IU/L or more are not uncommon.

- The plasma bilirubin rarely exceeds 200 µmol/L.

- Alkaline phosphatase activity is raised only slightly, if at all.

- Occasionally plasma amylase activities are increased due to underlying pancreatitis.

- Hypoglycaemia is a potential complication of severe liver damage.

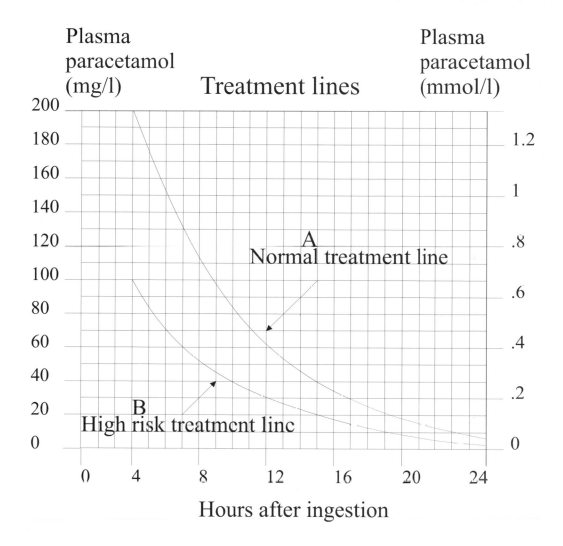

Figure 4.1. Paracetamol treatment line

- Measurement of the prothrombin time or INR is of greater clinical value than measurements of ALT and AST activity.

PLASMA CONCENTRATIONS
- A single plasma paracetamol concentration related to the time elapsed since ingestion, though not ideal, is currently the only method of adequately assessing the severity of a paracetamol overdose.

- The sample analysed should not be taken earlier than 4 hours after ingestion;

before that time absorption and distribution of the drug is incomplete and the result may be misleading.

- Two plasma concentrations separated by a few hours would probably give a better indication of prognosis but time restraints, particularly delays in presentation and the relatively short time window during which the antidotes are of maximum efficacy, render this impracticable. It may have a place in assessing staggered overdoses.

THE PARACETAMOL TREATMENT LINE (FIGURE 4.1)
- Was developed as a prognostic tool for identifying patients at risk of severe liver damage.

- Indicates patients at risk of developing ALT or AST activity >1000 IU/L – not fulminant hepatic necrosis and not life or death.

- 60% of patients with concentrations related to time above the conventional treatment line will develop an ALT or AST >1000 IU/L.

- The line is not infallible – 20% of patients below the conventional treatment line will develop an ALT/AST >1000 IU/L.

- The line was developed from observations in adults; its applicability to children is unknown, but there is no choice but to use it.

- Extrapolation of the line beyond 15 hours is unjustified – there are no data from untreated patients to support it.

- The line was developed from observations in adults who took paracetamol alone; its applicability to those who co-ingest opiate/opioid analgesics that delay gastric emptying is unknown, but there is no choice but to use it.

- The high risk line applies where microsomal oxidases may have been induced.

MANAGEMENT OF PATIENTS WHO PRESENT WITHIN 4 HOURS OF OVER-DOSE
- Gastric lavage if >150 mg/kg paracetamol has been ingested within the previous hour.
- Give a single dose of oral activated charcoal.

- Identify potential risk factors.

- Wait until 4 hours post-ingestion.

- At 4 hour post-ingestion take a blood sample for urgent plasma paracetamol concentration assess the risk of serious liver damage from the nomogram. Give N-acetylcysteine (NAC) if appropriate.

MANAGEMENT OF PATIENTS WHO PRESENT 4-8 HOURS AFTER OVERDOSE
- Gastric emptying and charcoal are of no value.

- Take a blood sample for urgent measurement of the plasma paracetamol concentration.

- Identify potential risk factors.

- Assess the risk of serious liver damage from the nomogram.

- Give NAC if appropriate.

MANAGEMENT OF PATIENTS WHO PRESENT >8 HOURS AFTER OVERDOSE
- Take a blood sample for urgent plasma paracetamol concentration.

- Start NAC immediately – clinicians should not wait for the plasma paracetamol result.

- Identify potential risk factors.

- Continue or stop NAC if the plasma paracetamol concentration related to time indicates risk or no risk respectively.

ASSESSMENT AT THE END OF NAC ADMINISTRATION
- Measure the prothrombin time or INR.

- Measure the plasma creatinine.

PARAQUAT

IMPORTANT FACTS

- Paraquat poisoning is now very uncommon in the UK.

- Ingestion is the most common route of absorption. Ingestion is associated with a high mortality though paraquat is poorly absorbed from the gut.

- The outcome and duration of survival after poisoning by ingestion are closely related to the quantity of paraquat ingested – the critical amounts are more than 6 g, 3-6 g and 1.5-3 g.

- Paraquat can be absorbed through skin. Rare fatalities have been reported but only after prolonged contact and in the presence of significant pre-existing dermal damage.

- Systemic poisoning does not occur after accidental inhalation of paraquat spray.

MECHANISMS OF TOXICITY

- Paraquat is actively accumulated by alveolar cells in the lungs, then undergoes redox cycling producing free radicals which cause lipid peroxidation that damages cells and impairs their function.

- Pulmonary fibrosis then develops.

CLINICAL FEATURES

The features and time course of poisoning vary according to the amount ingested:

Clinical feature of poisoning with paraquat		
>6 g ingested	**3-6 g ingested**	**1.5 - 3 g ingested**
Nausea	Nausea	Nausea
Vomiting	Vomiting	Vomiting
Abdominal pain	Salivation and hoarseness	Burns of the mouth,
Pallor	secondary to burns of the	tongue
Hypotension	mouth, tongue and larynx	Increasing breathless-
Acute pulmonary oedema	Acute renal failure	ness due to intra- and
Impaired consciousness	Increasing breathlessness due	inter-alveolar fibrosis
Convulsions	to haemorrhagic alveolitis	Death from respiratory
Death within 24-36 h	Death from respiratory failure	failure within 10-21
	within 5-7 days	days

LABORATORY FEATURES

- Evidence of acute renal failure.

- Mild hyperbilirubinaemia.

- Minor increases in the activity of alanine and aspartate aminotransferases.

- Hypoxaemia without hypercapnia.

SCREENING TESTS

URINE
- Urine voided within a few hours of ingestion is required.

- The urine is alkalinised by the addition of a small amount of sodium bicarbonate and a similar amount of sodium dithionite is then added. A colour varying from green to intense blue develops in the presence of paraquat; the more intense the blue colour, the higher the concentration of paraquat.

- This test is insensitive. Concentration using an ion-exchange resin has been advocated.

- A negative test on urine passed within 4 hours of alleged ingestion indicates that no significant quantity of paraquat has been absorbed.

- Paraquat is a 'hit and run' poison; the screening test will be negative if the urine tested was produced more than 4-6 hours post ingestion.

PLASMA
- The urine screening test described above can also be performed on 5 mL plasma but is unreliable.

PLASMA CONCENTRATIONS

- Are of value in determining the likely outcome of the incident and thus dealing with the patient's relatives and, occasionally, the patient.

- Concentrations are of no other value in management.

- Patients whose plasma paraquat concentrations fall above the line in Figure 4.2 at the relevant times after ingestion will almost certainly die regardless of treatment.

MANAGEMENT
- Treatment is entirely symptomatic and supportive.

- Activated charcoal may be more effective than gastric lavage in reducing absorption.

- Give anti-emetics if required.

- Analgesics and oral rinses are indicated for buccal burns.

- Give intravenous fluids to compensate for the inability to swallow and gastrointestinal fluid loss.

- Manage skin ulcers as burns.

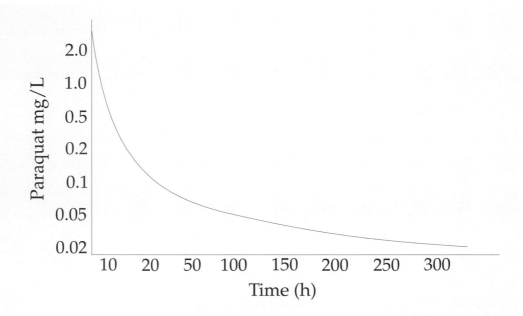

Figure 4.2. Plasma paraquat concentrations related to the time from ingestion. Patients who are above the line will almost certainly die and those below it survive.

- Avoid giving supplemental oxygen – it increases the risk of pulmonary damage.

- Currently available techniques cannot remove toxicologically significant quantities of paraquat.

- Corticosteroids, drugs to prevent free radical formation, free radical scavengers, immunosuppressive agents, radiotherapy to the lungs, or lung transplantation have not been shown to be of value.

PHENYTOIN

IMPORTANT FACTS
- Overdose may be therapeutic or due to intentional self-harm.

- Epileptics are those most likely to take deliberate overdoses of phenytoin.

MECHANISMS OF TOXICITY
- The mechanism is not understood.

- Toxic amounts of phenytoin have been shown to damage the cerebellar cortex in animals.

CLINICAL FEATURES

Clinical features of poisoning with phenytoin	
Common	**Uncommon**
Nausea	Coma
Vomiting	Convulsions
Nystagmus	
Inco-ordination	

LABORATORY FEATURES
- None of note.

PLASMA CONCENTRATIONS
- Therapeutic concentrations are within the range 8-15 mg/L (32-60 µmol/L).

- Measurement of plasma phenytoin concentrations is useful for confirming over- or under-dosage. The presence of nystagmus is a good indicator of a phenytoin concentration exceeding 30 mg/L (120 µmol/L).

- Monitoring of plasma concentrations post-overdose is important in deciding when to re-start regular treatment in an epileptic who has been phenytoin toxic.

MANAGEMENT
- Gastric lavage for patients who present within one hour of ingestion of a substantial overdose.

- Multiple-dose oral activated charcoal may increase elimination.

QUININE

IMPORTANT FACTS

- Quinine overdose is usually accidental in children and deliberate in adults.

- In the UK today, the availability of quinine is due to it being prescribed to treat night cramps in elderly patients.

- Abroad, quinine still has an important role as an antimalarial drug.

- Severe and irreversible visual impairment is the major long-term hazard of poisoning.

- Quinine and quinidine are optical isomers.

MECHANISMS OF TOXICITY

- The mechanism underlying oculotoxicity of quinine is not known.

- The cardiotoxicity of quinine is due to membrane stabilising effects.

CLINICAL FEATURES – ACUTE

Cinchonism is the term used to describe the collective common features of quinine intoxication. (Quinine was first isolated from the bark of the cinchona tree.)

Clinical features of acute poisoning with quinine	
Common	**Uncommon**
Nausea	Convulsions
Vomiting	Coma
Tinnitus	ECG abnormalities including QT- and later
Impaired hearing	QRS-interval prolongation
Blurred vision leading to	Ventricular tachycardia
blindness	Cardiac arrest

CLINICAL FEATURES – CHRONIC

- Tunnel vision (i.e. visual field constriction) may be a long-term complication and may be so severe that some patients will qualify to be registered as blind.

LABORATORY FEATURES

- None of note.

PLASMA CONCENTRATIONS

- Knowledge of the plasma quinine concentration is of prognostic value but does not aid management of acute poisoning.

- Visual impairment is likely with plasma quinine concentrations exceeding 10 mg/L.

- Cardiac complications are likely with plasma quinine concentrations greater than 15 mg/L.

MANAGEMENT

- Gastric lavage for patients who present within one hour of ingestion of a substantial overdose.

- A single dose of oral activated charcoal may be given to reduce absorption.

- Multiple-dose oral activated charcoal enhances the elimination of quinine.

- Stellate ganglion block and systemic vasodilators are ineffective.

- Cardiovascular disturbances are managed appropriately.

SALICYLATES

IMPORTANT FACTS
- Salicylate poisoning, usually with aspirin (acetylsalicylic acid), remains common, although much less so than in the 1960s and 70s.

- Poisoning with methyl salicylate is rare, but potentially much more serious.

- Continued absorption of aspirin from the GI tract is common after initial hospital treatment.

- Sustained release salicylate formulations may adhere to form concretions (known as bezoars or pharmacobezoars) in the stomach leading to prolonged continuing absorption.

- Significant intoxication can result from the application of salicylate-containing ointments to abnormal skin e.g. 5% salicylic acid to remove the scales of psoriasis.

- Significant intoxication can result from the repeated application of salicylate-containing teething gels to the gums of infants.

- Salicylate poisoning is a potential cause of a high anion gap acidosis.

- Chronic salicylism is uncommon in the UK but may present with unusual features, particularly in the elderly.

Dose/toxicity relationships in salicylate poisoning	
Dose of salicylate mg/kg	**Toxicity**
150	mild
250	moderate
750	severe/fatal

However, these correlations must be regarded only as guidelines; the amount stated to have been ingested is frequently unreliable.

MECHANISMS OF TOXICITY
- There are direct effects on the inner ear.

- There are direct effects on the GI tract.

- The respiratory centre is stimulated.

- Salicylates uncouple oxidative phosphorylation.

- As plasma salicylate concentrations increase, metabolism becomes saturated and elimination of salicylate becomes increasingly dependent on urinary excretion.

- Salicylates are weak acids – a normal or low arterial hydrogen ion concentration (normal or high pH) keeps them ionised and prevents them distributing to tissues, particularly the brain.

CLINICAL FEATURES

Salicylism is the term used to describe the collective common features of salicylate intoxication.

Clinical features of salicylism	
Common	**Uncommon**
Nausea	Impaired consciousness
Vomiting	Delirium
Vasodilatation	Pulmonary oedema
Sweating	Renal failure
Tinnitus	Convulsions
Impaired hearing	Arrhythmias
Acid-base disturbances	

LABORATORY FEATURES

- Hypokalaemia and hyperkalaemia have been reported.

- Hypoglycaemia is a possible, but rare, complication.

- There may be prolongation of the prothrombin time or INR, but it is minor and of no clinical importance.

- It is widely held that the initial acid-base disturbance of salicylate intoxication is a respiratory alkalosis which is superseded by dominant metabolic acidosis; the evidence for this sequence is debatable.

- Children under the age of four years commonly present with acidaemia secondary to a dominant metabolic acidosis.

- Older children (over the age of four years) and adults often have a mixed respiratory alkalosis and metabolic acidosis resulting in a normal arterial hydrogen ion concentration (pH) or alkalaemia if the respiratory effect dominates.

- Adults occasionally develop acidaemia with a dominant metabolic component – such patients are at increased risk of pulmonary oedema and death.

- Hypocalcaemia is a potential complication of urinary alkalinisation.

PLASMA SALICYLATE CONCENTRATIONS
- In general, clinical features correlate poorly with plasma salicylate concentrations.

- Patients with the common features of salicylism (see above) are likely to have plasma salicylate concentrations exceeding 300 mg/L (2.2 mmol/L).

- The mortality in patients with plasma salicylate concentrations exceeding 700 mg/L (5.1 mmol/L) is about 5%.

- Repeat plasma salicylate concentrations may be needed because of slow and continuing absorption of the drug.

MANAGEMENT
- Gastric lavage for patients who present within one hour of ingestion of a substantial overdose.

- Multiple-dose oral activated charcoal may enhance the elimination of salicylate as well as reduce its absorption.

- Measure the plasma salicylate concentration.

- Children with plasma salicylate concentrations <350 mg/L (2.5 mmol/L) do not require specific treatment.

- Adults with plasma salicylate concentrations <450 mg/L (3.3 mmol/L) do not require specific treatment.

- Urine alkalinisation (achieved with intravenous infusion of sodium bicarbonate) is indicated for children and adults with plasma salicylate concentrations exceeding 350 mg/L (2.5 mmol/L) and 450 mg/L (3.3 mmol/L) respectively.

- Forcing a diuresis is of no therapeutic value and should not be attempted – it is potentially lethal in acidaemic patients and those with neurological features.

- Serious consideration should be given to the urgent use of haemodialysis in patients with plasma salicylate concentrations >700 mg/L (5.1 mmol/L).

- Patients with life-threatening intoxication (usually with CNS features) should be given intravenous glucose since neuroglycopenia may occur in the absence of hypoglycaemia.

SELECTIVE SEROTONIN REUPTAKE INHIBITORS

IMPORTANT FACTS
- This group of comparatively new antidepressants includes citalopram, fluoxetine, fluvoxamine, paroxetine and sertraline.

- Poisoning with them is increasingly common as they replace the tricyclic antidepressants.

MECHANISM OF TOXICITY
- As the group name indicates, selective serotonin reuptake inhibitors (SSRIs) block the reuptake of serotonin at synapses in the CNS, thus increasing the amounts of transmitter in these areas.

CLINICAL FEATURES
The SSRIs are considerably less toxic in overdose than the tricyclic antidepressants.

Clinical features of poisoning with SSRIs	
Common	**Uncommon**
Nausea	Convulsions
Vomiting	Bradycardia
Agitation	Junctional rhythm
Tremor	
Drowsiness	
Sinus tachycardia	

LABORATORY FEATURES
- Raised creatine kinase activity.

PLASMA CONCENTRATIONS
- Are of no value in the management of poisoning.

MANAGEMENT
- Commonly, no specific treatment is required.

- Supportive measures should be instituted as necessary.

SMOKE INHALATION

IMPORTANT FACTS
- Inhalation of smoke from fires kills more people than do flames.

- Smoke is a complex mixture of particles and toxic gases some of which, unlike heat, reach the alveoli where they are absorbed.

- The nature of the gases present in smoke depends on the materials that are burning and the temperature of combustion; carbon monoxide, hydrogen cyanide, isocyanates, phosgene, acrolein and a variety of aldehydes may all be generated.

- Domestic fires are often the consequence of individuals falling asleep often while under the influence of alcohol or drugs.

MECHANISMS OF TOXICITY
- Heat damage to the respiratory tract is uncommon below the level of the larynx.

- Many of the gases produced in fires reach the alveoli, damaging them and impairing gas exchange.

- Carbon monoxide reduces the oxygen-carrying capacity of the blood and oxygen delivery to tissues.

- Hydrogen cyanide prevents oxygen utilisation by cells.

- The role of inhaled particles (mainly carbon) in the pathogenesis of pulmonary lesions has not yet been elucidated.

- Pre-existing chronic obstructive pulmonary disease increases the morbidity from smoke inhalation.

CLINICAL FEATURES

Clinical features of smoke inhalation	
Common	**Uncommon**
Nausea	Respiratory depression
Burns may or may not be present	Hypotension
Eyes may be streaming	Pulmonary oedema
A metallic taste in the mouth	Coma
Sore throat	
Hoarseness	
Cough	
Production of sputum containing soot particles	
Wheeze	
Breathlessness and chest tightness	
Cyanosis	
Tachycardia	

LABORATORY FEATURES
- Hypoxaemia is often much more severe than would be suspected from the symptoms and signs unless oxygen has been given by the emergency services on the way to hospital.

- $PaCO_2$ is usually slightly reduced, reflecting hyperventilation.

- Arterial hydrogen ion concentration varies depending on whether hypoxia has been of sufficient severity and duration to produce a metabolic acidosis.

- Elevated blood cyanide concentrations are commonly found but are seldom toxic.

BLOOD CONCENTRATIONS
- Carboxyhaemoglobin concentrations are commonly in the range 10-50%.

- Concentrations on arrival at hospital may underestimate the severity of exposure due to the combination of dissociation when exposure stops and oxygen administration on the way to hospital.

- Blood cyanide concentrations are occasionally high but cannot be assayed in an emergency.

MANAGEMENT

- The victim will have been removed from the smoke by the emergency services.

- A clear airway and adequate ventilation is essential.

- The oxygen content of the inspired air should be increased as far as possible.

- Carry out arterial blood gas analysis.

- Measure the carboxyhaemoglobin concentration.

- Laryngoscopy or fibreoptic bronchoscopy may be required to determine the full extent of the damage to the respiratory tract.

- Carbon monoxide poisoning should be managed as described above (p63).

- The possibility of concomitant cyanide poisoning should be considered if patients fail to respond.

- Do not give cyanide antidotes to stable patients – they are inherently toxic and may make matters worse rather than better.

THEOPHYLLINE

IMPORTANT FACTS
- Most theophylline formulations available in the UK are of a modified release type; absorption may therefore be slow.

- Patients on modified release type preparations should be kept on the same brand to minimise the risk of toxicity.

- Both therapeutic excess and massive overdose can cause life-threatening toxicity.

- There is no validated system for classifying the severity of theophylline intoxication.

MECHANISMS OF TOXICITY
- Stimulates ATPase.

- Inhibits phosphodiesterase.

- Causes hyperinsulinaemia and increases circulating catecholamines shifting potassium from the extracellular fluid into cells causing hypokalaemia.

- The profound and rapid change in potassium across the membranes of cardiac myocytes may be an important factor in the genesis of arrhythmias.

CLINICAL FEATURES
Slow absorption may delay the onset of features of toxicity for up to 12 hours after ingestion.

Clinical features of poisoning with theophylline	
Common	**Uncommon**
Nausea	Haematemesis
Vomiting	Seizures
Abdominal pain	Hyperthermia
Agitation	Supraventricular and ventricular tachycardias
Tremor	Coma
Sinus tachycardia	Rhabdomyolysis
Ectopic beats	
Hypotension	

LABORATORY FEATURES
- Hypokalaemia.

- Hyperglycaemia.

- Glycosuria.

- Elevated circulating insulin concentrations.

- Metabolic acidosis.

PLASMA CONCENTRATIONS
- Therapeutic theophylline concentrations are in the range 10-20 mg/L (55-110 µmol/L).

MANAGEMENT
- Gastric lavage for patients who present within one hour of ingestion of a substantial overdose.

- Multiple-dose oral activated charcoal is of critical importance since gut dialysis may be as efficient as charcoal haemoperfusion in enhancing the elimination of theophylline.

- Monitor the plasma potassium concentration at short intervals.

- Measure the plasma glucose concentration.

- Carry out arterial blood gas analysis in patients showing any evidence of serious toxicity.

- Measure the plasma theophylline concentration urgently. In asymptomatic patients, four or more hours post ingestion.

- Anti-emetics should be given – the commonly used, less expensive ones such as cyclizine are often ineffective – ondansetron is usually effective.

- Replace fluid (including blood) lost through vomiting.

- Correct hypokalaemia in the belief that it is the rapid change in the potassium gradient across excitable membranes that is the mechanism of important cardiac and neurological toxicity.

- Control convulsions if necessary.

- In non-asthmatic patients, administration of β-adrenoceptor blocking drugs may reduce tachycardia.

- Correct metabolic acidosis if appropriate.

- Continue to monitor potassium concentrations during recovery, particularly if potassium supplements have been given – rebound hyperkalaemia is to be expected.

THYROXINE

IMPORTANT FACTS
- Thyroxine is most likely to be ingested in excess by young children.

- Toxic features seldom develop.

- Overdose of other thyroid hormones is rare.

MECHANISMS OF TOXICITY
- Thyroxine (T4) is converted to the active hormone T3.

- Thyroxine stimulates all aspects of metabolism.

CLINICAL FEATURES
The onset of symptoms is usually delayed until 3-6 days after ingestion.

Clinical features of poisoning with thyroxine	
Common	**Uncommon**
Agitation	Ocular features of hyperthyroidism
Irritability	Sweating
Hyperactivity	Altered bowel habit
Sinus tachycardia	Atrial fibrillation
Increased respiratory rate	Thyroid storm
Pyrexia	
Dilated pupils	

LABORATORY FEATURES
- None, other than the effects on thyroid hormone concentrations (see below).

PLASMA CONCENTRATIONS
- Plasma T4 and T3 concentrations increase to many times normal.

- TSH concentrations fall.

MANAGEMENT
- Gastric lavage for patients who have ingested more than 2 mg of thyroxine and present within one hour.

- A single dose of oral activated charcoal may be given.

- Measure plasma T4 and T3 concentrations in a blood sample taken 6-12 hours after ingestion.

- Patients with normal results will not develop toxic features and require no further intervention.

- Review patients with high T4 concentrations 4-5 days after ingestion; those who show evidence of thyroid overactivity should be given propranolol for 5 days.

TRICYCLIC ANTIDEPRESSANTS

IMPORTANT FACTS
- Tricyclic antidepressant poisoning is becoming less common as they are being replaced by newer antidepressants, particularly the selective serotonin reuptake inhibitors.

- Tricyclic antidepressants remain an important cause of suicide by drugs.

MECHANISMS OF TOXICITY
- Tricyclic antidepressants block the reuptake of noradrenaline into peripheral and intracerebral neurones so increasing local concentrations of monoamines.

- They have anticholinergic effects.

- They also show class 1 antiarrhythmic activity.

CLINICAL FEATURES

Clinical features of poisoning with tricyclic antidepressants	
Common	**Uncommon**
Drowsiness	Coma – particularly lasting longer than 24 hours
Dry mouth	Increased muscle tone
Dilated pupils	Hyperreflexia
Sinus tachycardia	Extensor plantar responses
	Convulsions
	Urinary retention
	Skin blisters
	Rhabdomyolysis
	Hypothermia
	Respiratory depression
	Decreased myocardial contractility leading to hypotension
	Cardiac conduction abnormalities
	Ventricular tachycardia and fibrillation

LABORATORY FEATURES
- Include those of respiratory depression, metabolic acidosis and possible rhabdomyolysis.

PLASMA CONCENTRATIONS
- Are of no value in the management of acute poisoning.
- Concentrations exceeding 1 mg/L are associated with severe toxicity.

MANAGEMENT
- Gastric lavage for patients who present within one hour of ingestion of a substantial overdose.

- Give a single dose of oral activated charcoal.

- Most patients recover with supportive therapy alone.

- Optimum oxygenation, control of convulsions and correction of acidosis is the most appropriate method of managing cardiotoxicity.

- Give adults with serious cardiotoxicity sodium bicarbonate (50 mmol intravenously over 20 minutes) even if there is no acidosis.

- Use lignocaine for ventricular tachycardia that is compromising cardiac output.

- Physostigmine salicylate, a cholinesterase inhibitor, has no role as an antidote in tricyclic poisoning.

- Do not use flumazenil in combined tricyclic antidepressant/benzodiazepine overdose – it may uncover tricyclic antidepressant-induced convulsions.

- Use oral or intravenous diazepam to sedate patients who are delirious and have auditory and visual hallucinations during recovery.

- Elimination techniques are of no value.

VOLATILE SUBSTANCE ABUSE

IMPORTANT FACTS
- Volatile solvent abuse (VSA) is the currently accepted term for what was previously called 'glue sniffing'.

- VSA is the intentional inhalation of any of a variety of volatile organic chemicals contained in products such as such as solvents, glues, aerosols and fuels.

- The chemicals commonly involved are butane (cigarette lighter refill fluid), chlorofluorocarbons (aerosols), long-chain hydrocarbons (petrol), chlorinated hydrocarbons, n-hexane and toluene (glues).

MECHANISMS OF TOXICITY
- The effects of VSA are similar to those of ethanol.

- Initially the CNS is stimulated but is then depressed by further exposure.

- Sensitivity of the myocardium to endogenous catecholamines is increased leading to arrhythmias.

CLINICAL FEATURES
The features found in any given individual depend to some extent on the chemical involved. There may be both psychological and physical consequences of long-term VSA in addition to the better-known acute effects.

Acute effects
The clinical features of intoxication with volatile substances are similar to those of alcohol intoxication with initial CNS stimulation followed by depression. Sudden death from cardiac arrest is not uncommon, this may be related to the current prevalence of butane as a propellant.

Chronic psychological features
- Dependence on VSA.

- Unexplained listlessness.

- Moodiness.

- Psychotic symptoms.

Clinical features of volatile substance abuse	
Common	**Uncommon**
Euphoria	Hallucinations
Excitement	Coma
Blurred vision	Convulsions
Dysarthria	Status epilepticus
Unsteadiness	Cardiac arrhythmias
Feelings of omnipotence	Rhabdomyolysis
Impaired judgement	'Glue-sniffer's rash' (red spots around the
Irritability	mouth and nose)
Headache	Cerebral oedema
Antisocial behaviour	Pulmonary oedema
Deliberate self-harm	Jaundice (chlorinated hydrocarbons)
	Renal tubular necrosis

- Poor performance at school.

LONG-TERM PHYSICAL FEATURES
- Loss of appetite.

- Weight loss.

- Motor and sensory peripheral neuropathy (hexane, toluene).

- Encephalopathy (toluene, tetraethyl lead in petrol).

- Cerebellar degeneration.

LABORATORY FEATURES
- Metabolic acidosis.

- Hypokalaemia.

- Hyperchloraemia.

- Hypophosphataemia.

- Features secondary to rhabdomyolysis.

- Distal renal tubular acidosis.

PLASMA CONCENTRATIONS
- Are of no value in the management of VSA.

MANAGEMENT (ACUTE POISONING)
- Remove the person from further exposure.

- VSA intoxication is usually short-lived and does not require treatment.

- It may be necessary to 'talk down' or sedate excited or agitated patients.

- Ensure a clear airway, adequate respiration and cardiac output if poisoning is severe.

- Other measures as necessitated by clinical developments.

FURTHER READING

ALTERNATIVE MEDICINES
Shannon M. Alternative medicines toxicology: a review of selected agents. J Toxicol Clin Toxicol 1999; **37:** 709-13.

AMPHETAMINES AND ECSTASY
Boot BP, McGregor LS, Hall W. MDMA (ecstasy) neurotoxicity: assessing and communicating the risks. Lancet. 2000; **355:** 1818-21.

Ernst T, Chang L, Leonido-Yee M, Speck O. Evidence for long-term neurotoxicity associated with methamphetamine abuse. A[1]H MRS study. Neurology 2000; **54:** 1344-9.

ANTICOAGULANTS
Casner PR. Superwarfarin toxicity. Am J Therap 1998; **5:** 117-20.

Baglin T. Management of warfarin (coumarin) overdose. Blood Reviews 1998; **12:** 91-8.

McCarthy PT, Cox AD, Herrington DJ, Evely RS, Hampton E, Al-Sabah AI, Massey E, Jackson H, Ferguson T. Covert poisoning with difenacoum: clinical toxicological observations. Hum Exper Toxicol 1997; **16:** 166-70.

BENZODIAZEPINES
Hojer J, Baehrendtz S, Gustafsson L. Benzodiazepine poisoning: Experience of 702 admissions to an intensive care unit during a 14-year period. J Intern Med 1989; **226:** 117-22.

CARBAMATE INSECTICIDES
Wagner S. Diagnosis and treatment of organophosphate and carbamate intoxication. Occup Med (Philadelphia) 1997; **12:** 239-49.

CARBAMAZEPINE
Apfelbaum JD, Caravati EM, Kerns WP 2nd, Bossart PJ, Larsen G. Cardiovascular effects of carbamazepine toxicity. Ann Emerg Med 1995; **25:** 631-5.

Montoya-Cabrera MA, Sauceda-Garcia JM, Escalante-Galindo P, Flores-Alverez E, Ruiz-Gomez A. Carbamazepine poisoning in adolescent suicide attempters. Effectiveness of multiple-dose activated charcoal in enhancing carbamazepine elimination. Arch Med Res 1996; **27:** 485-9.

CARBON MONOXIDE
Weaver LK. Hyperbaric oxygen in carbon monoxide poisoning. Brit Med J 1999; **319:** 1083-4.

International Programme on Chemical Safety. Environmental Health Criteria 213. Carbon monoxide, 2nd ed. World Health Organisation, Geneva, 1999.

CARDIAC GLYCOSIDES
Kinlay S, Buckley NA. Magnesium sulfate in the treatment of ventricular arrhythmias due to digoxin toxicity. J Toxicol Clin Toxicol 1995; **33:** 55-9.

Williamson KM, Thrasher KA, Fulton KB, La Pointe NM, Dunham GD, Cooper AA, Barrett PS, Patterson JH. Digoxin toxicity: an evaluation in current clinical practice. Arch Intern Med 1998; **158:** 2444-9.

COCAINE
Blaho K, Logan B, Winberry S, Park L, Schwilke E. Blood cocaine and metabolite concentrations, clinical findings and outcome of patients presenting to an ED. Ann J Emerg Med 2000; **18:** 593-8.

Hatsukami D, Fischman MW. Crack cocaine and cocaine hydrochloride – are the differences myth or reality? J Am Med Ass 1996; **276:** 1580-8.

Marzuk PM, Tardiff K, Leon AC, Hirsch CS, Stajic M, Portera L, Hartwell N, Iqbal MI. Fatal injuries after cocaine use as a leading cause of death among young adults in New York city. New Engl J Med 1995; **332:** 1753-7.

Rubin RB, Neugarten J. Medical complications of cocaine: changes in pattern of use and spectrum of complications. J. Toxicol Clin Toxicol 1992; **30:** 1-12.

The biological basis of cocaine addiction. Ed: Quinones-Jenab V. Ann NY Acad Sci 2001; **937.**

ETHANOL
Ernst AA, Jones K, Bick TG, Sanchez J. Ethanol ingestion and related hypoglycemia in a pediatric and adolescent emergency department population. Acad Emerg Med 1996; **3:** 46-69.

ETHYLENE GLYCOL
Barceloux DG, Krenzelok EP, Olson K, Watson W. American Academy of Clinical Toxicology Practice Guidelines on the Treatment of Ethylene Glycol Poisoning. Ad

Hoc Committee. J Toxicol Clin Toxicol 1999; **37:** 537-60.

Brent J, McMartin K, Phillips S, Burkhart KK, Donovan JW, Wells M, Kulig K. Fomepizole for the treatment of ethylene glycol poisoning. New Engl J Med. 1999; **340:** 832-8.

HYDROFLUORIC ACID
Dunn BJ, MacKinnon MA, Knowlden NF, Billmaier DJ, Derelanko MI, Rosch GM, Naas DJ, Dahlgren RR. Topical treatments for hydrofluoric acid dermal burns. Further assessment of efficacy using an experimental pig model. J Occup Environ Med 1996; **38:** 507-14.

HYPOGLYCAEMIC DRUGS
Palatnick W, Meatherall RC, Tenenbein M. Clinical spectrum of sulfonylurea overdose and experience with diazoxide therapy. Arch Intern Med 1991; **151:** 1859-62.

Roberge RJ, Martin TG, Delbridge TR. Intentional massive insulin overdose: recognition and management. Ann Emerg Med 1993; **22:** 228-34.

IRON SALTS
Chyka PA, Butler AY, Holley JE. Serum iron concentrations and symptoms of acute iron poisoning in children. Pharmacotherapy 1996; **16:** 1053-8.

Tenenbein M. Benefits of parenteral deferoxamine for acute iron poisoing. J Toxicol Clin Toxicol 1996; **34:** 485-9.

LEAD
Lifshitz M, Hashkanazi R, Phillip M. The effect of 2, 3 dimercaptosuccinic acid in the treatment of lead poisoning in adults. Ann Med 1997; **29:** 83-5.

LITHIUM
Scharman EJ. Methods used to decrease lithium absorption or enhance elimination. J Toxicol Clin Toxicol 1997; **35:** 601-8.

MERCURY
O'Carroll RE, Masterton G, Dougall N, Ebmeier KP, Goodwin GM. The neuropsychiatric sequelae of mercury poisoining. The Mad Hatter's disease revisited. Br J Psychiat 1995; **167:** 95-8.

Torres-Alanis O, Garza-Ocanas L, Pineyro-Lopez A. Intravenous self-administration of metallic mercury: report of a case with a 5 year follow-up. J Toxicol Clin Toxicol

1997 **35:** 83-7.

METHANOL
Brent J, McMartin K, Phillips S, Aaron C, Kulig K. Fomepizole for the treatment of Methanol Poisoning. New Engl J Med. 2001; **344:** 424-9.

Jacobsen D, McMartin KE. Antidotes for methanol and ethylene glycol poisoning. J Toxicol Clin Toxicol 1997; **35:** 126-43.

OPIATE AND OPIOID ANALGESICS
Weinbroum A, Rudick V, Sorkine P, Nevo Y, Halpern P, Geller E, Niv D. Use of flumazenil in the treatment of drug overdose: a double-blind and open clinical study in 110 patients. Crit Care Med 1996; **24:** 199-206.

ORGANOPHOSPHATE INSECTICIDES
Thiermann H, Mast U, Klimmek KR, Eyer P, Hibler A, Pfab R, Felgenhauer N, Zilker T. Cholinesterase status, pharmacokinetics and laboratory findings during obidoxime therapy in organophosphate poisoned patients. Hum Exper Toxicol 1997: **16:** 473-80.

Wagner SL. Diagnosis and treatment of organophosphate and carbamate intoxication. Occup Med (Philadelphia) 1997; **12:** 239-49.

QUININE
Mackie MA, Davidson J, Clarke J. Quinine – acute self poisoning and ocular toxicity. Scot Med J 1997; **42:** 8 -9.

Nordt SP, Clark RF. Acute blindness after severe quinine poisoning. Am J Emerg Med 1998; **16:** 214-5.

PARACETAMOL
Vale JA, Proudfoot AT. Paracetamol (acetaminophen) poisoning. Lancet 1995; **346:** 547-52.

NEUROLEPTIC MALIGNANT SYNDROME
Adnet P, Lestavel P, Krivosic-Horber R. Neuroleptic malignant syndrome. Br J Anaesth 2000; **85:** 129-135.

PAEDIATRIC PESTICIDE POISONING
Thompson JP. Suspected paediatric poisoning in the UK, I and II Hum Exp Toxicol 1994; **13:** 529-33 and 534-6.

POISONING IN THE ELDERLY
Klein-Schwartz W, Oderda GM. Poisoning in the elderly. Epidemiological, clinical and management considerations. Drugs Aging 1991; **1:** 67-89.

SALICYLATES
Chapman BJ, Proudfoot AT. Adult salicylate poisoning: Deaths and outcome in patients with high plasma salicylate concentrations. Quart J Med 1989; **72:** 699-707.

Phillips S, Brent J, Kulig K, Heiligenstein J, Birkett M. Fluoxetine versus tricyclic anti-depressants: a prospective multicenter study of antidepressant drug overdoses. J Emerg Med 1997; **15:** 439-45.

SELECTIVE SEROTONIN RE-UPTAKE INHIBITORS
Gross R, Dannon PN, Lepkifker E, Zohar J, Kotler M. Generalized seizures caused by fluoxetine overdose. Am J Emerg med 1998; **16:** 328-9.

SMOKE INHALATION
Orzel RA. Toxicological aspects of fire smoke: polymer pyrolysis and combustion Occup Med 1993; **8:** 415-29.

Shusterman D, Alexeeff G, Hargis C, Kaplan J, Sato R, Gelb A, Becker C, Benowitz N, Gillen M, Thollaug S, Balmes J. Predictors of carbon monoxide and hydrogen cyanide exposure in smoke inhalation patients. J Toxicol Clin Toxicol 1996; **34:** 61-71.

THEOPHYLLINE
Minton NA, Henry JA. Acute and chronic human toxicity of theophylline. Hum Exper Toxicol 1996; **15:** 471-81.

THYROXINE
Hack JB, Leviss JA, Nelson JS, Hoffman RS. Severe symptoms following massive intentional L-thyroxine ingestion. Vet Hum Toxicol 1999; **41:** 323-6

TRICYCLIC ANTIDEPRESSANTS
Buckley NA, Dawson AH, Whyte IM, Henry DA. Greater toxicity in overdose of dothiepin than of other tricyclic antidepressants. Lancet 1994; **343:** 159-62.

Taboulet P, Michard F, Muszynski J, Galliot-Guilley M, Bismuth C. Cardiovascular repercussions of seizures during cyclic antidepressant poisoning. J Toxicol Clin Toxicol 1995; **33:** 205-11.

VOLATILE SUBSTANCE ABUSE

Ramsey J, Taylor J, Anderson HR, Flannagan RJ. Volatile substance abuse in the United Kingdom. NIDA Res Monogr 1995; **148:** 205-49.

Chapter 5

Illustrative cases of acute poisoning

CASE 1

HISTORY
An 18 year-old male presented to the Accident and Emergency Department at 09.10h claiming to have taken some 'painkiller tablets' around tea-time the previous day. He complained of nausea, vomiting, dizziness and abdominal cramps but was other-wise normal. Blood was taken for electrolytes, renal function tests, full blood count, INR, paracetamol and salicylate.

COMMENT
• Paracetamol would be high on the list of drugs that he may have taken.

• Given that the overdose may have been taken 16 hours ago, it would be consistent with current practice to start N-acetylcysteine infusion before the plasma paracetamol result becomes available.

• Note that measurement of salicylate has also been requested though the presentation does not suggest it. Because occasionally some overdoses of painkillers are mixed, intervention can be effective and concentrations easily measured, it is common practice for clinical biochemistry laboratories to measure paracetamol and salicylate at the same time.

INVESTIGATIONS
The laboratory results were as follows:

Na^+ mmol/L	K^+ mmol/L	Urea mmol/L	Creatinine μmol/L	Paracetamol mmol/L	Salicylate mmol/L
149	3.6	12.1	95	0.43 (65 mg/L)	<0.05 (<7 mg/L)

INR	H^+ nmol/L	pH	pCO_2 KPa	pO_2 KPa	HCO_3^- mmol/L
1.6	40	7.40	4.8	14.1	30

COMMENT
- The elevated urea but normal creatinine are consistent with dehydration due to vomiting.

- While a hypochloraemic alkalosis might be anticipated as a result of vomiting, any tendency to alkalosis is countered by a mild metabolic acidosis commonly seen in paracetamol poisoning.

- The paracetamol concentration is above the treatment line. The efficacy of N-acetylcysteine declines rapidly at this time after ingestion and treatment should be continued.

- The INR is slightly prolonged suggesting liver damage has already been sustained and is likely to increase.

- INR is the most sensitive of the readily available tests for hepatic function.

HISTORY 2
The patient developed a rash soon after the NAC infusion was started and also volunteered the information he was an epileptic.

COMMENT
- Adverse reactions to N-acetylcysteine are common.

- Cessation of the infusion for a short time and recommencement at a lower infusion rate is usually all the treatment that is required.

- Oral methionine would not be an option as the patient is vomiting.

- Hepatic enzyme inducing drugs, including some anticonvulsants or chronic excess intake of ethanol, predispose to greater risk of paracetamol toxicity (roughly double) due to induction of hepatic microsomal enzymes.

- NAC therapy in this scenario should minimise hepatic damage. The liver will regenerate to give normal function provided there are no further insults.

CASE 2

HISTORY

On a hot summer day a 26 year-old farm worker sprayed some crops with malathion. At the end of the day he felt anxious and restless, had a headache and was sweating. He also had a red rash on his trunk and face. On examination he was found to have hypersalivation and miosis.

COMMENT

- The subject has organophosphate poisoning.

- Exposure has been due to failure to wear protective clothing.

- The patient's clothes should be removed.

- Blood should be taken for red cell cholinesterase measurement.

- Treatment with atropine and pralidoxime is not indicated immediately, but may be in the next few hours.

INVESTIGATIONS

The plasma cholinesterase was 18% of normal.

COMMENT

- Both RBC and plasma cholinesterases are decreased in organophosphate poisoning.

- RBC cholinesterase is depressed for longer than plasma cholinesterase following organophosphate poisoning.

- Some organophosphates (e.g. malathion) inhibit plasma cholinesterase to a greater extent than the red cell enzyme.

- The farm worker's plasma cholinesterase activity is consistent with moderate poisoning.

- As exposure was percutaneous, systemic toxicity manifested itself slowly and avoidance of worsening toxicity must be considered. This was achieved by continued therapy and repeated washing of the exposed area.

- Cold water washing is preferred initially as cutaneous absorption may be enhanced by warm/hot water.

- Supportive treatment is provided as required.

- Atropine antagonises the effects of acetylcholine.

- The degree to which red cell and plasma cholinesterase activity is inhibited is a guide to severity of the poisoning.

- Carbamates form short-lived reversible complexes with cholinesterase while organophosphates form longer lasting complexes.

- Enzyme activity is recoverable provided the subject receives pralidoxime before the complex 'ages'.

CASE 3

HISTORY

A 51 year-old male with a history of depression presented to hospital. He had nausea and vomiting and on examination was found to be ataxic. Shortly after he had a fit, following which his Glasgow Coma Score was 9. He was also hyperventilating and had tachycardia. The results of laboratory investigations were as follows:

Na$^+$ mmol/L	K$^+$ mmol/L	Urea mmol/L	Creatinine μmol/L	H$^+$ nmol/L	pCO$_2$ kPa	pO$_2$ kPa	HCO$_3^-$ mmol/L
133	5.2	8.2	135	80	2.2	13.0	4

COMMENT

There is a partly compensated metabolic acidosis, the cause of which is not immediately apparent.

INVESTIGATIONS

Glucose mmol/L	Chloride mmol/L	Calcium (adjusted) mmol/L	Phosphate mmol/L
15.3	80	1.57	0.87

COMMENT

• Glucose is raised by stress.

• The low calcium is suspicious and suggested complex formation.

• A measurement of serum osmolality is required.

FURTHER INVESTIGATIONS

The serum osmolality was 391 mosm/Kg.

COMMENT

• The calculated osmolality (see p18 for the formula) is 299 mmol/L; the osmolar gap is therefore 92 mosm/kg.

• This is a high anion gap metabolic acidosis.

• The presence of hypocalcaemia suggests ethylene glycol poisoning is the most likely cause for the illness though fluoride is a possibility.

- A high index of suspicion may be needed to reach the correct diagnosis in a poisoned patient.

TREATMENT
The patient was immediately started on intravenous ethanol in dextrose and blood sent for analysis to confirm ethylene glycol poisoning.

COMMENT
- The patient requires careful biochemical monitoring.

- As the hypocalcaemia is caused by complexation of calcium with oxalate, a metabolite of ethylene glycol, the hypocalcaemia needs urgent correction.

OUTCOME
The ethylene glycol result was available two hours later with a concentration of 5.8 g/L. The patient had deteriorated with renal failure and proteinuria and a Glasgow Coma Score of 4. As attempts were being made to arrange haemodialysis the patient suffered a cardiorespiratory arrest and died.

COMMENT
- Unfortunately if there is no clear history it is not easy to detect ethylene glycol ingestion.

- Ethanol competitively inhibits the metabolism of ethylene glycol preventing the production of further acidic metabolites but those already present are not removed.

- Urgent haemodialysis while continuing to administer ethanol and calcium will yield the best result.

- The clinical biochemist is in a good position to have a high index of suspicion when confronted with the marked biochemical abnormalities that typify this poisoning.

- Despite life-saving intervention being achievable, delay in diagnosis often means that patients die because appropriate therapy has not been given.

- 4-methylpyrazole is now available on a named patient basis and is to be preferred as ethanol contributes to the sedation and acidosis.

CASE 4

HISTORY
A 58 year-old businessman was found slumped in his car with a hosepipe leading from the exhaust to the interior. He was admitted to hospital. He was hypotensive, had a tachycardia, and had irregular deep respirations with some cyanosis. 100% oxygen was administered.

Na$^+$ mmol/L	K$^+$ mmol/L	Urea mmol/L	Creatinine µmol/L	Glucose mmol/L
139	5.8	9.1	155	7.8

H$^+$ nmol/L	pCO$_2$ kPa	pO$_2$ kPa	COHb %	(on oxygen)
55	4.1	25.0	78	

COMMENT
- Carbon monoxide binds to haemoglobin causing a left shift in the oxygen dissociation curve; the affinity for haemoglobin is 250 times greater than that of oxygen.

- Reduction of cardiac output and, consequently, of tissue perfusion results in anaerobic metabolism and a metabolic acidosis, but also hypoxaemia with a reduced arterial oxygen content.

INVESTIGATIONS
The carboxyhaemoglobin level one hour later was 55%.

COMMENT
- The COHb concentration is consistent with significant morbidity and a fatal outcome.

OUTCOME
90 minutes after admission the patient died of cardiorespiratory arrest without regaining consciousness.

COMMENT
- The decrease in oxygen availability exacerbates any pre-existing atherosclerotic reduction in myocardial oxygen supply and thus older patients are more liable

to die. Patients who survive may have demonstrable persistent intellectual deficits.

- The half-life of COHb breathing air is around 4 to 5 hours and is reduced to 90 minutes on 100% oxygen.

- Hyperbaric oxygen reduces the half-life of COHb to 20 minutes.

- Use of hyperbaric oxygen is still controversial and only available in a very few centres. Patients at particular risk (see p64) should be considered for referral for hyperbaric oxygen; this should be discussed with the National Poisons Information Service.

- Access to hyperbaric oxygen presents serious logistical problems. Such services are usually associated with the off-shore oil industry or navy rather than national health services, administrative arrangements are time-consuming, the distance to the nearest chamber may be considerable and it may be difficult to arrange the staff required to accompany the patient.

CASE 5

HISTORY

A 78 year-old woman accompanied her 8 year-old grandson to hospital after the child had swallowed 'some of her heart tablets'. The precise number was not known. The child was pale, confused, vomiting and hypotensive. He had a bradycardia of 38 beats/min. He weighed 32kg.

Na+ mmol/L	K+ mmol/L	Urea mmol/L	Creatinine μmol/L	Digoxin μg/L
137	6.2	5.1	73	12.5

COMMENT

- The hyperkalaemia with a high serum digoxin indicates that this is a severe overdose.

- Digoxin binds to receptors blocking Na/K-ATPase action and causing increased intracellular sodium and increasing extracellular potassium. The bradycardia may progress to sinus arrest.

TREATMENT

The medical team decide to use digoxin-specific Fab fragment antibodies.

COMMENT

- An estimate of the body load of digoxin can be obtained using the formula:

$$\frac{SDC \times 5.6 \times body\ weight}{1000}$$

(Where SDC is the serum digoxin concentration in μg/L, the value of 5.6 in the numerator is the volume of distribution of digoxin in litres and body weight is in kg. The 1000 in the denominator converts the load to mg).

- In this case the load is therefore:

$$\frac{12.5 \times 5.6 \times 32}{1000} = 2.24\ mg$$

- The body load must be multiplied by 64 to obtain the weight of Fab fragments required.

- The amount of Fab required is therefore 143 mg.

- Fab fragments are very expensive.

CASE 6

HISTORY
A previously fit and well 18 year-old female was brought to hospital by her friends at 04.00h. They had been to a dance club. After some time she was found dazed and confused in the toilets. She had since become stuporose.

Na$^+$ mmol/L	K$^+$ mmol/L	Urea mmol/L	Creatinine μmol/L	Glucose mmol/L
107	3.6	2.1	51	6.3

Urine Na$^+$ mmol/L	Serum osmolality mosm/kg	Urine osmolality mosm/kg
28	230	336

COMMENT
- She has severe dilutional hyponatraemia with inappropriate urine concentration.

- She is young and healthy, significant renal disease is excluded and adrenal and thyroid disease are unlikely.

- 0.5L of 1.8% saline was infused and frusemide given 8 hours later.

INVESTIGATIONS
She was not known to be taking any prescribed medication. A drug screen was performed later that morning.

Screen negative: opiates, cannabis, benzodiazepines and cocaine.
Screen positive: methamfetamine.

COMMENT
- Immunoassay screens lack specificity for amfetamines.

- Definitive identification of the amfetamine compound involved will be required.

- It is a reasonable conclusion that this is a hyponatraemia secondary to excess water intake after using ecstasy.

FURTHER INVESTIGATIONS
Repeat investigations after saline infusion gave the following results:

Na⁺ mmol/L	K⁺ mmol/L	Urea mmol/L	Creatinine μmol/L	MDMA identified in urine
121	6.5	3.6	65	

COMMENT
- Rapid correction of hyponatraemia is usually contra-indicated, however in this case the onset was also rapid.

- Correction of hyponatraemia together with fluid restriction once consciousness has been regained should result in full recovery.

- Dilutional hyponatraemia occurs because dancers are aware of the malignant hyperthermia syndrome (with rhabdomyolysis and a high mortality rate) that arises in dance clubs if inadequate amounts of water are taken.

- Water was promoted as a counter to malignant hyperthermia syndrome but current harm reduction advice advocates isotonic fluids.

- Treatment is not dependent on the drug screen result.

CASE 7

HISTORY
A 16 year-old boy ingested the contents of a sachet of paraquat granules following a tiff with his girlfriend. He presented at hospital the following day complaining of nausea and vomiting. No abnormalities were noted on examination and his serum urea and electrolytes and full blood count were normal. He was admitted for observation but took his own discharge. Ten days later he presented complaining of breathlessness and a chest x-ray showed areas of fibrosis. He was admitted but the fibrosis progressed over the next three weeks when he died in respiratory failure.

COMMENT
- Ingestion of a sachet (~ 2g) of granular paraquat is sufficient to cause death.

- With such amounts there are few symptoms initially.

- Higher doses reflect the corrosive nature of liquid paraquat formulations with renal damage.

- If patients survive long enough irreversible damage to the lungs caused by the free radical action of paraquat leads to death from hypoxia.

INVESTIGATIONS
On admission, about 15 hours post-ingestion, his serum paraquat was 0.3 mg/L.

COMMENT
- The paraquat prognostic curve suggests a poor outcome.

- There is no known effective treatment for paraquat poisoning.

- Knowledge of the prognosis is helpful to the patient and relatives to enable them to prepare themselves.

- The alkaline dithionite urine test has a high false negative rate and should be interpreted with caution.

- The test may be improved by using an anion exchange resin to increase sensitivity.

CASE 8

HISTORY
A 48 year-old scientific instrument engineer restored and repaired old scientific gauges for a hobby. He conducted his hobby in an old hut in which he had a paraffin heater. One winter he complained of weight loss, weakness and flu-like illness and depression. Neurological examination revealed muscle weakness and wasting with incoordination.

Na$^+$ mmol/L	K$^+$ mmol/L	Urea mmol/L	Creatinine µmol/L
132	5.2	12.7	175

COMMENT
- Gauges often contain elemental mercury.

- Elemental mercury is not toxic when ingested.

- Spillage of elemental mercury on to floors results in inhalation of mercury vapour.

- Exposure to mercury vapour is increased in closed, heated environments.

- Spillages onto the floor and the build up of heat in the hut are likely to have resulted in high atmospheric mercury concentrations.

INVESTIGATIONS
A urine sample was examined for mercury and a result of 180 nmol/mmol creatinine was found.

COMMENT
- Removal from this environment was sufficient to ensure that the patient recovered.

- He was advised to work in a contained area with air extraction in future.

- Acceptable Health and Safety urinary mercury concentrations are below 40 nmol/mmol creatinine.

- Removal from exposure is often sufficient treatment in mercury poisoning, although a chelating agent such as dimercaprol may be used to rapidly reduce the body load.

- Elemental mercury is lipophilic and, once absorbed, forms inorganic complexes which lead to organ damage.

- Mercurous salts (Hg^+) are less toxic than mercuric (Hg^{2+}) or alkyl mercury compounds.

CASE 9

HISTORY
A 23 year-old was admitted with a sinus tachycardia of 115 beats/min following ingestion of her siblings theophylline capsules. She had increased muscle tone. The following laboratory results were obtained from a blood sample taken on admission.

Na⁺ mmol/L	K⁺ mmol/L	Urea mmol/L	Creatinine µmol/L	Glucose mmol/L	Theophylline µmol/L
140	2.4	7.0	105	12.1	295

(Therapeutic range 50-110 µmol/L)

COMMENT
• The hypokalaemia and hyperglycaemia are typical of theophylline overdose reflecting increased catecholamine activity.

• The theophylline concentration is consistent with mild poisoning.

• As she was a smoker it was decided no active intervention was necessary; smokers clear theophylline twice as fast as non-smokers.

• Arterial blood gases should be checked as there may be a metabolic acidosis.

• The hypokalaemia is due to intracellular shift and if potassium supplementation has been given there may be rebound hyperkalaemia as the poisoning resolves.

FURTHER INVESTIGATIONS
She later developed tremor and flap. A further urgent theophylline measurement was performed and the concentration found to be 790 µmol/L (12 hours post-admission).

COMMENT
• Theophylline overdose must be regarded with the utmost seriousness; life-threatening toxicity develops insidiously.

• The commonest theophylline formulations are of a slow-release type.

• After overdose, therefore, it may take 12-24 hours for the full extent of the poisoning to be revealed.

- Prompt administration of activated charcoal helps minimise absorption.

- Whole bowel irrigation may also be effective in minimising absorption of slow-release preparations.

- Multiple-dose oral charcoal is less problematic to use and is the treatment of choice provided vomiting can be controlled.

- Failing multiple-dose oral charcoal, severe theophylline toxicity may require the use of charcoal haemoperfusion.

- Plasma theophylline concentrations may rebound after haemoperfusion is stopped.

CASE 10

HISTORY
A 30 year-old man arrived at the Accident and Emergency Department in a taxi. He was hallucinating, violent, paranoid and too dangerous to approach for a blood sample. After an hour he collapsed and was thought to have had a myocardial infarction. Blood taken at that point showed:

Na+ mmol/L	K+ mmol/L	Urea mmol/L	Creatinine µmol/L	Glucose mmol/L	CK U/L	AST U/L	CKMB (mass)
144	4.9	10.1	110	8.3	7200	127	4%

COMMENT
- The elevated urea and normal creatinine are consistent with pre-renal uraemia.

- The CK and CKMB results indicate skeletal muscle damage and probable rhabdomyolysis.

- Despite having evidence of early renal failure and rhabdomyolysis, both of which would raise the serum potassium, the latter is normal indicating that potassium release from damaged cells is being counterbalanced by movement into healthier cells.

OUTCOME
His respiration was failing and he was admitted to the Intensive Care Unit where he continued to deteriorate with uncontrollable convulsions that made respiratory support difficult. One seizure resulted in cardio-respiratory arrest from which he could not be revived. Subsequent discussion with the taxi driver revealed he had collected the patient from the airport. At post mortem the patient was found to have been a 'body-packer' transporting cocaine into the country. The bags of cocaine were each wrapped in three condoms but, despite this, some had leaked.

COMMENT
- Even confirming cocaine as the cause of the patient's clinical features would not have enabled any effective intervention other than emergency laparotomy, although whole gut irrigation might have been useful.

- Given the condition of the patient it is debatable whether the outcome would have been different. The lethal oral dose of cocaine is 1-1.5 g, thus only one package need leak for death to occur.

Chapter 6

Forensic toxicology

Analytical forensic toxicology is typically performed by specialist forensic laboratories with access to a wide range of instrumentation. Clinical laboratories are most likely to be involved in cases performed for the Coroner (Procurator Fiscal in Scotland). The analyst is acting on behalf of the pathologist to enable him to establish whether a poison was the cause of death. In a Coroner's Court there is no need to consider intention nor to provide evidence for criminal proceedings though the results may be referred to in court.

Forensic toxicology in the UK is performed either in university departments of forensic medicine, police laboratories or the Forensic Science Service. There are also specialist private laboratories. Much of the work in forensic science is related to documents, serology, DNA testing, fabrics, paints, firearms etc.

In relation to illegal substances the emphasis is on examination of seizures made by police and customs i.e., determining whether material is an illegal substance, and by examining its composition, where it is likely to have originated from.

Forensic toxicology covers the spectrum of examining the deceased in an aircraft accident for carboxyhaemoglobin to determine whether they had died because of the fire or the crash, to determining whether a poison has caused a sudden death in a previously fit individual, or was an individual under the influence of drugs or alcohol at the time of an offence.

As there are clear legal implications in forensic toxicology the documentation procedures are more rigorous than for clinical samples.

SAMPLES

The pathologist should take blood samples from sites which are clearly identified, the femoral vein is a preferred site as well as cardiac blood. The ability to do this depends on the amount of decomposition. Urine may not be available. Sections of organs, particularly liver, but also heart and brain, may also be made available. Decomposition can be extensive and consequently there may be no formed elements in blood. Products of decomposition e.g. putrescine and cadaverine make the analytical challenge more difficult as they may interfere in the assays masking or mimicking drugs. Assays that are suitable for clinical toxicology may not, therefore, be appropriate for forensic toxicology. Methods used in forensic toxicology need to be validated for that purpose; enzyme based assays may have high backgrounds or suffer inhibition, chromatographic methods suffer interfering peaks and matrix retention effects. Extraction efficiencies may also be compromised.

Analysis of tissue requires that it be liquefied as the first stage in preparation; this used to be done by homogenisation in perchloric acid but the harsh chemical and mechanical conditions result in the loss of the compound of interest or poor recovery. The use of proteases e.g. subtilisin which digest the proteins, greatly enhances recovery and the mild conditions minimise analyte loss; the resulting liquid can then be processed using standard techniques.

DOCUMENTATION

In forensic cases it is clearly necessary to be able to offer incontrovertible evidence that the analyses referred to in court are demonstrably from the examined subject; a similar requirement applies to coroner's and procurator fiscal cases. Consequently Chain of Custody procedures are utilised (Figure 6.1).

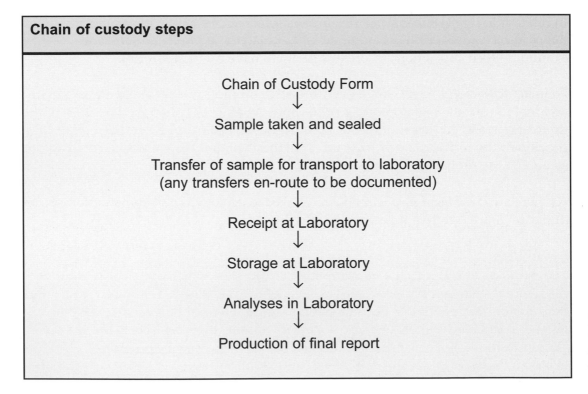

Chain of custody steps

Chain of Custody Form
↓
Sample taken and sealed
↓
Transfer of sample for transport to laboratory
(any transfers en-route to be documented)
↓
Receipt at Laboratory
↓
Storage at Laboratory
↓
Analyses in Laboratory
↓
Production of final report

Figure 6.1. Chain of custody steps (a signature is required at each step)

As the term implies, chain of custody is provision of proof that a sample has progressed in a fully traceable way from its origin to final analysis and report; that all actions relating to the transport, storage, analysis and report collation are identifiable and that as a consequence it is possible to be sure beyond reasonable doubt that (a) the sample came from the subject, (b) there is no possibility of contamination or exchange of the sample.

This is achieved by taking a sample from the subject and labelling with their identification and sealing the cap with evidential tape. If the subject is alive then their countersignature to the chain of custody form is usually advised. As the sample is transferred from the pathologist or police surgeon onwards via transportation to receipt at the laboratory, those passing on and receiving the sample should sign, date and time their actions. The process continues once the sample is in the laboratory until the final report is prepared.

ANALYSIS

Methods to be used for forensic toxicology work should have documented standards of performance in terms of accuracy, precision, sensitivity etc. Sometimes a court may require an analyst to describe to the court how an analysis was performed, what the possibilities of error are and their qualifications to perform such analyses. It is clearly important that those directing such activities are satisfied as to the standards applied to the analysis.

Given the large number of compounds that need to be considered in addition to interferents, especially post-mortem decomposition products, a single analysis may not be sufficient to provide definitive identification of the presence of a substance and, therefore, confirmation using a technique based on a different analytical principle is commonly required.

The analytical strategy may be informed by the history, or the exclusion of certain substances requested. A common requirement is to detect whether a poison has contributed to death, since a history may be unhelpful or non-existent. In such circumstances a screening strategy is utilised; frequently an immunoassay 'frontline' is used due to its simplicity.

Compounds with similar physico-chemical structures and/or behaviour may behave similarly in a given analytical mode e.g. chromatography, immunoassay. The likelihood of similar behaviour in both systems is low, but not impossible. Historically the definitive technique has been seen as gas-chromatograpy-mass-spectrometry; the former providing separation (i.e. purity) and the latter definitive molecular information as well as sensitivity. As not all compounds will volatilize or chromatograph well, derivatisation with agents such as trimethylsilylesters has been used. However, newer techniques such as gas-chromatography-tandem mass-spectrometry, or liquid-chromatography-mass spectrometry or even tandem mass-spectrometry alone offer simpler, definitive and sensitive analytical options to the forensic toxicologist.

Forensic toxicology does not readily lend itself to quality assurance, especially external quality assurance. It is easy to see how blood alcohol measurement may be controlled; breath alcohol meters have their own internal checking procedure. There have been international collaborative surveys in which case histories plus samples were circulated, with very mixed results, but adequate matrix and appropriate drugs and metabolites to service other than a very few laboratories is very difficult to achieve. For these reasons external quality assurance schemes (EQAS) do not exist for forensic toxicology analyses, and though specialist services (e.g. the Forensic Science Service) have their own, they are closed schemes. The UK National External Quality Assurance Scheme for Drug Assays is based on blood ethanol and carboxy-haemoglobin concentrations, but does run a toxicology case scheme in which about one-third of cases are 'forensic', generally samples are of non-decomposed fluids. The lack of generally available 'true' EQAS makes the use of good internal quality control vital to enable proof of good performance.

REPORTING

Having been satisfied that the results are qualitatively and quantitatively accurate the reporter has to collate the analytical, clinical and scientific information available to reach a judgement on the significance of the result in the context of the case. The report should reflect the certainties and uncertainties of the findings and give an indication of the probable contribution of the findings to the circumstances of the case. The report must be signed by a responsible analyst.

There is an increasing awareness of the difficulty of interpreting drug concentrations post-mortem. Drugs which are widely distributed i.e. bound, are released during decomposition, and there is a tendency to equilibration as barriers to osmosis become more permeable, i.e. while there may be no discernable change in macro structures, there are changes at the cellular level. The consequence is an increase in concentrations in post-mortem blood; these increases may be several-fold greater than ante-mortem levels. Thus, individuals on therapeutic doses of drugs with concentrations ante-mortem consistent with the therapy may have greatly increased post-mortem blood concentrations. The situation is further complicated by there being differences according to the site from which the blood was sampled. Cardiac blood may be significantly different from femoral vein blood; the latter best reflects ante-mortem levels. The degree of change relates to the degree of post-mortem change, the ambient temperature, the drug in question and the position of the body. In addition to these complications, much of the literature values before the mid 1970's are based on inaccurate methods with poor, variable recovery from post-mortem material, particularly tissue. Reference to valid data needs to be performed. Cases that have to go to court are time consuming. Forensic laboratories have Reporting Officers who are trained in giving evidence and whose role is the presentation of facts and uncertainties in cases which may often hinge on the forensic evidence. This is clearly very different from the circumstances a clinical toxicologist would be familiar with. Evidence presented at a coroner's court is intended to enable the Coroner (Procurator Fiscal) to determine the significance of poisoning as a contributing factor to the cause of death.

It is beyond the scope of this monograph to provide information on the custody and presentation of evidence and the reader should refer to books on forensic jurisprudence. It is, however, important to recall that the evidence given is to the court and is not on behalf of either the defence or the prosecution. The aim is to provide a balanced and fair judgement based on the evidence. The expert witness must establish their credentials to the court and are expected to give an opinion if qualified to do so. The individual offering such services must be aware of the time required for such activities.

FURTHER READING

Forrest AR. Forensic Toxicology ACP Broadsheet no. 137: April 1993. Obtaining samples at post mortem examination for toxicological and biochemical analyses.

Chapter 7

Substance abuse testing

Substance abuse (SA) can be considered in four categories:-

(a)   Legal
(b)   Workplace
(c)   Clinical
(d)   Sports

Each has different requirements; the first has been partially considered in the previous section. Workplace testing incorporates employment and pre employment screening. Clinical SA testing may be in the management of poisoning or as part of a rehabilitation programme. Sports SA testing is to ensure no performance enhancing drugs have been taken.

NEEDS OF THE SERVICE

LEGAL TESTING

Tests resulting in prosecution of an offender or offered as defence for a crime are only part of the picture. Challenges between relatives over child safety are not uncommon. Substance misusers tend not to agree to testing if they would test positive, but may be required to be tested by a Court. Such individuals may also seek testing if they have been abstinent and by demonstrating this on testing regain access to their children. Testing of inmates of prisons is performed to enable control of illegal substances in prison: this is more successful if there is a rehabilitation programme in place.

WORKPLACE TESTING

Practised in the U.S. for many years, workplace testing is now more prevalent in Europe. Companies test prospective and current employees to detect users who will be on a contract requiring them to declare substance dependency. A positive sample with no declaration is grounds for instant dismissal. In some occupations testing is mandatory for safety reasons e.g. fixed terminus transport systems such as in air or rail travel the pilot or driver must be tested by law.

CLINICAL

Use of illegal substances is not necessarily a clinical problem. However, as with legal drugs there may be adverse reactions, some of which may result in death, which have to be considered. Three categories can be considered: acute presentation due to toxicity, consequence of the impurities in illegal substances and the mode of introduction of the substances. The illegality of the drugs, their addictive potential and their effects combine to result in significant social dysfunction and a frequently chaotic lifestyle which, allied to the risk of infection from HIV and Hepatitis in this group, gives them a mortality rate around ten times greater than for their non-drug using peers.

The most successful policy in combating this situation is harm-reduction. Harm-reduction aims, through the provision of needle exchange, structured methadone replacement therapy, free condoms and educational efforts, to stabilise users behaviour with the aim of eventually weaning the user off drugs completely.

SPORTS
Governing bodies, e.g. the International Olympic Committee, agree lists of drugs that may be considered performance enhancing and must not be used by competitors on pain of disqualification and suspension.

ANALYTICAL REQUIREMENTS

LEGAL
Legal challenges should be dealt with under chain of custody procedures. The implications of positive and negative results are the same as workplace testing (see below). Urine tests only demonstrate abstinence over a period of 2-3 days for most abused substances. The detection of drugs in hair, particularly opiates, which extends over one or two months is more convincing. Claims for sweat and saliva as better matrices still await validation, but the latter is becoming increasingly used. These are currently only available in a very few specialist centres.

WORKPLACE
Prospective employees and employees whose contract or legislation demands it undergo SA testing. The implications of a false positive to the individual could self-evidently be devastating; equally an employer may be put at risk if there is a false negative.

To ensure positives are genuine the approach in this testing is to use chain of custody, with gas-chromatography-mass-spectrometry confirmation. Any less than this is open to effective challenge.

Screening cut-offs used are those advised by European testing guidelines, the screens are performed by immunoassay for those drugs in Figure 7.1, confirmation is at a lower concentration. There are no agreed cut-off values for other drugs. The American Substance Abuse Mental Health Services Agency (SAMHSA), formerly NIDA, recognise the poppy seed defence and require morphine to be >2000 mg/L and a 6 mono-acetylmorphine >10 mg/L to be found before a positive opiate result is reported.

SPORTS

Anabolic steroid abuse is not uncommon amongst those whose sport requires a good physique. In sports the definition of what substances are illegal in the context of competition is defined by the Sport's ruling body.

Such testing is performed by specialised laboratories well practised in the art of a 'total' service e.g. the International Olympic Committee fund a specialised laboratory in each member country.

Urine Screen cut-off concentrations for abused substances				
Substance	Main metabolite	Detection time	Screening (µg/L)	Confirmation (µg/L)
Marijuana	Δ^9tetrahydro-cannabinolic acid	2-4 weeks	50	15
Heroin	Morphine	2-3 days	300	50
Cocaine	Benzoylecognine	1 – 2 days	300	50
Amfetamine		1 – 2 days	300	300
Benzodiazepines		1 – 2 days	300	300

Figure 7.1. Urine screen cut-off concentrations for abused substances

LIABILITY

Those undertaking any form of SA testing must be appropriately indemnified. Thus clinical testing may be part of the normal service of a clinical laboratory and indemnity for errors would be through the employing authority and possibly the Medical Defence Union or Medical Protection Society. However, workplace, legal or sports testing need to be performed to even higher standards with attention to detail. Any legal actions for errors may well be against the individual as well as the employer; if the employer is an NHS Trust then it is unlikely they could provide indemnity from their contingency fund and indeed may be acting *ultra vires* if they do. The situation on this point is not clear: anyone intending embarking on this would be well advised to obtain clarification.

OCCUPATIONAL AND ENVIRONMENTAL TOXICOLOGY

Occupational exposure to toxic substances is subject to the Health & Safety at Work Act and the various Regulations enforced by the Health and Safety Executive (HSE). Monitoring of exposure may well be by air sampling or by monitoring biological fluids; analyses are offered through the HSE Laboratories.

Two main topic areas are heavy metal exposure and pesticides. While laboratory support may be required to investigate acute exposure, this is rarer than monitoring chronic exposure which may be a necessary part of ensuring that toxicity for individuals in the workplace is avoided.

Monitoring may be required, for example, of exposure to mercury, lead or cadmium in electroplating or smelting operation or of farm workers using pesticides. The monitoring of serum and erythrocyte cholinesterase is a marker of exposure to organophosphorous compounds.

A high index of suspicion of occupational or environmental poisoning is required to enable detection.

FURTHER READING

HERBAL POISONS
De Smet PA, van den Ertwegh AJ, Lesterhuis W, Stricker BH. Hepatotoxicity associated with herbal tablets Brit Med J 1996; **313:** 92.

But PP, Tomlinson B, Cheung KO, Yong SP, Szeto ML, Lee CK. Adulterants of herbal products can cause poisoning. Brit Med J 1996; **313:** 117.

GAMMA HYDROXY BUTYRATE
Timby N, Eriksson A, Bostrum K. Gamma-hydroxybutyrate associated deaths. Am J Med 2000; **108:** 518-9.

METHADONE
Ward J, Hall W, Mattick RP. Role of maintenance treatment in opioid dependence. Lancet. 1999; **353:** 221-6.

Hendra TJ, Gerrish SP, Forrest ARW. Lesson of the Week: Fatal methadone overdose. Brit Med J. 1996; **313:** 481-2.

MERCURY
Satoh H. Occupational Health and environmental toxicology of mercury and its compounds. Ind Health 2000; **38:** 153-64.

OPIATES
Farrell M, Neelman J, Griffiths P, Strang J. Suicide and overdose among opiate addicts. Addiction. 1996; **91:** 321-3 (Editorial).

Darke S, Ross J, Hall W. Overdose among heroin users in Sydney, Australia I and II Addiction 1996; **91:** 405-11 and 413-7.

Index